OXFORD MEDICAL PUBLICATIONS

Pulmonary Hypertension

Oxford Specialist Handbooks published and forthcoming

General Oxford Specialist Handbooks

A Resuscitation Room Guide
Addiction Medicine
Day Case Surgery
Hypertension
Perioperative Medicine,
Second Edition
Postoperative Complications,
Second Edition
Renal Transplantation

Oxford Specialist Handbooks in Anaesthesia

Anaesthesia for Emergency Care
Cardiac Anaesthesia
Neuroanaesthesia
Obstetric Anaesthesia
Ophthalmic Anaesthesia
Paediatric Anaesthesia
Regional Anaesthesia, Stimulation and
Ultrasound Techniques
Thoracic Anaesthesia

Oxford Specialist Handbooks in Cardiology

Adult Congenital Heart Disease
Cardiac Catheterization and
Coronary Intervention
Cardiac Electrophysiology and
Catheter Ablation
Cardiovascular Computed
Tomography
Cardiovascular Magnetic Resonance
Echocardiography, Second Edition
Fetal Cardiology
Heart Failure
Hypertension
Inherited Cardiac Disease
Nuclear Cardiology
Pulmonary Hypertension
Valvular Heart Disease

Oxford Specialist Handbooks in Critical Care

Advanced Respiratory
Critical Care

Oxford Specialist Handbooks in End of Life Care

End of Life Care in Cardiology
End of Life Care in Dementia
End of Life Care in Nephrology
End of Life Care in Respiratory
Disease
End of Life in the Intensive
Care Unit

Oxford Specialist Handbooks in Neurology

Epilepsy
Parkinson's Disease and
Other Movement Disorders
Stroke Medicine

Oxford Specialist Handbooks in Paediatrics

Paediatric Dermatology
Paediatric Endocrinology
and Diabetes
Paediatric Gastroenterology,
Hepatology, and Nutrition
Paediatric Haematology and
Oncology
Paediatric Intensive Care
Paediatric Nephrology, Second
Edition
Paediatric Neurology, Second Edition
Paediatric Radiology
Paediatric Respiratory Medicine

Oxford Specialist Handbooks in Pain

Spinal Interventions in Pain
Management

Oxford Specialist Handbooks in Psychiatry

Child and Adolescent Psychiatry
Forensic Psychiatry
Old Age Psychiatry

Oxford Specialist Handbooks in Radiology

Interventional Radiology
Musculoskeletal Imaging
Pulmonary Imaging
Thoracic Imaging

Oxford Specialist Handbooks in Surgery

Cardiothoracic Surgery
Colorectal Surgery
Hand Surgery
Hepatopancreatobiliary Surgery
Neurosurgery
Operative Surgery, Second Edition
Oral Maxillofacial Surgery
Otolaryngology and Head and
Neck Surgery
Paediatric Surgery
Plastic and Reconstructive Surgery
Surgical Oncology
Urological Surgery
Vascular Surgery

Oxford Specialist Handbooks
Pulmonary Hypertension

Clive Handler

Consultant in Pulmonary Hypertension,
Royal Free Hospital, London,
Honorary Senior Lecturer in Medicine,
University College London,
Honorary Consultant Cardiologist,
Guy's and St Thomas' Hospitals,
London, UK

Gerry Coghlan

Consultant Cardiologist,
Royal Free Hospital,
London, UK

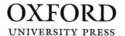

OXFORD
UNIVERSITY PRESS

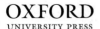

OXFORD
UNIVERSITY PRESS

Great Clarendon Street, Oxford, OX2 6DP,
United Kingdom

Oxford University Press is a department of the University of Oxford.
It furthers the University's objective of excellence in research, scholarship,
and education by publishing worldwide. Oxford is a registered trade mark of
Oxford University Press in the UK and in certain other countries

© Oxford University Press 2012

The moral rights of the authors have been asserted

First Edition published in 2012
Impression: 1

British Library Cataloguing in Publication Data

Data available

Library of Congress Cataloging in Publication Data

Data available

ISBN 978-0-19-957256-4

Printed in China by
C&C Offset Printing Co. Ltd

Foreword

The medical and economic burden of pulmonary hypertension has grown considerably in recent years. Thanks to major advances in its understanding and management, this condition no longer remains an enigma to many clinicians. Previously considered as an orphan disease, that is, a condition which affects few individuals and is overlooked by the medical profession and pharmaceutical companies, the concept that pulmonary hypertension is overlooked cannot be considered to be the case today. We have indeed progressed a long way since 1973 when the WHO sponsored the first international meeting on a mysterious condition named 'primary pulmonary hypertension', a few years after a frightening outbreak of hundreds of cases was observed in Switzerland, Austria, and Germany in subjects exposed to the aminorex diet pill. Since then, world pulmonary hypertension conferences have been organized in 1998 (Evian, France), 2003 (Venice, Italy), and 2008 (Dana Point, California, USA) and the most recent set of European guidelines have been jointly published by the European Society of Cardiology and the European Respiratory Society in 2009. The fifth world symposium on pulmonary hypertension will take place in 2013 in Nice, France. At this occasion international experts in the field will review the whole spectrum of pulmonary hypertension, covering basic and clinical science.

Therefore, *Pulmonary Hypertension* by Clive Handler and Gerry Coghlan from the Royal Free Hospital, London, is very timely and the authors should be congratulated for the quality of their work which elegantly summarizes major information on a fast-growing field. This manuscript is nicely illustrated and very pleasant to read. Healthcare professionals from various backgrounds, researchers, and medical students will better understand and approach this condition based on the valuable information summarized in this book.

Marc Humbert, MD, PhD

Paris, June 2012

Preface

Pulmonary arterial hypertension (PAH) is a rare and serious condition of unknown cause and associated with a wide variety of medical conditions. The prognosis of patients with PAH is similar to some forms of advanced cancer. It is characterized by a progressive increase in pulmonary vascular resistance leading to right ventricular failure and premature death. Its prevalence ranges from 15–50 patients per million population with an relatively young average age of 45 years.

PAH can be diagnosed only by right heart catheterization (RHC) showing a mean pulmonary artery pressure (mPAP) ≥25mmHg with a normal pulmonary capillary wedge pressure (PCWP) of ≤15mmHg (pre-capillary PH). This haemodynamic state may also be caused by various lung diseases: interstitial lung disease, chronic obstructive pulmonary disease, chronic thromboembolic disease, pulmonary hypertension, and, less commonly, a variety of haematological, systemic, and metabolic conditions.

Post-capillary pulmonary hypertension (PH) is a comparatively much more common haemodynamic state when the mPAP ≥25mmHg and the PCWP ≥16mmHg. Common causes include various heart diseases (systolic and/or diastolic impairment due to systemic hypertension, coronary heart disease, or valvular problems).

It is important to distinguish PAH from PH by RHC because treatment of PH depends on the cause; PAH specific treatments are contraindicated in post-capillary PH.

This book focuses on adult PAH which is classified according to aetiology into idiopathic (the commonest type of PAH); heritable; drugs and toxins; and associated causes which include a wide variety of medical conditions (connective tissue diseases, HIV, portal hypertension, congenital heart disease, schistosomiasis, and chronic haemolytic anaemias).

PAH is also associated with a diverse group of medical conditions of unclear or multifactorial mechanisms; haematological disorders, e.g. haemolytic anaemias, myelproliferative disorders, splenectomy, systemic disorders (sarcoidosis, histiocytosis, neurofibromatosis); metabolic disorders (glycogen storage disease, Gaucher disease, thyroid disorders); and others: (tumoural obstruction of the pulmonary arteries, fibrosing mediastinitis, chronic renal failure on dialysis).

The pathological changes in all types of PAH are similar: medial hypertrophy, intimal proliferation, fibrosis and vasoconstriction affect the small distal pulmonary arteries. There are also complex lesions (plexiform and dilated lesions) and thrombosis. These abnormalities increase the pulmonary vascular resistance and lead to right ventricular failure and death.

The clinical presentation of PAH depends on its severity and its effects on right ventricular function. Exertional breathlessness, fatigue, and weakness are the early symptoms but are non-specific and may occur in several other more common conditions. Unless PAH is considered or suspected on echocardiography, diagnosis and treatment are delayed. PAH should be considered and investigated in cases of unexplained breathlessness.

The time from symptom onset to diagnosis remains lamentably long, often 2 years or more, due to lack of awareness of the condition and its rarity compared to other causes of breathlessness.

Treatments which do not affect the underlying pathological processes are referred to as 'supportive'. They include anticoagulation to reduce the increased risk of thromboembolism, diuretics to control symptomatic oedema due to right heart failure, digoxin as a weak inotrope, and oxygen to correct hypoxaemia.

Treatments which target the pathogenetic abnormalities of PAH, are called 'disease specific' or 'targeted' therapies. There are three classes of drugs which target three of the pathways implicated in PAH: prostacyclin and prostanoids; endothelin receptor antagonists; and phosphodiesterase-5 inhibitors. Compared to most cardiac and respiratory drugs, they are expensive; annual costs range from £4500 for sildenafil, £20,000 for ERAs, and £32,000 for prostacyclin and its analogues, excluding the cost of drug delivery devices. New drugs are being evaluated in randomized controlled trials (RCTs).

The duration of most of the trials of each of these classes of PAH-targeted therapies has been only 3–4 months. None of the trials have been designed to evaluate the effects of these drugs on mortality and so it is difficult to draw conclusions about long-term effects. In the short term, the drugs appear promising with improvements in functional class and 6-minute walk distance (6MWD) by 35–55m. They appear to promote clinical stability and symptom improvement. There is no evidence that one group of drugs or one member of a group is superior.

A recent meta-analysis of 23 RCTs showed a 38–43% decrease in all-cause mortality. There was a 61% reduction in hospitalizations in the treated patients compared to patients randomized to placebo. The trials were not powered to analyse survival or long-term outcomes.

Until 10 years ago, before the use of PAH targeted treatments, median survival of IPAH from the time of diagnosis was 2.8 years. Survival at 1, 3, and 5 years was 68%, 48%, and 24% respectively. Registry data suggest that survival for IPAH and other types of PAH has improved over the last few years since the availability of new treatments.

Prostanoids are usually reserved for patients in World Health Organization (WHO) class IV because they are usually given intravenously with attendant risks of infection.

Although the quality of life and outlook for PAH patients remains grim, the promising results of these drugs have encouraged PAH clinicians and patients by providing short-term benefits and, in some patients, stabilization of the disease, but more effective drugs are urgently required.

The role of combination therapies, using more than one PAH-specific therapy, appears logical as it attacks more than one pathogenetic pathway simultaneously. There is some evidence from RCTs that combination therapy slightly improves exercise capacity and time to clinical worsening, but no evidence that it improves mortality. Add-on combination therapy improves 6MWD by 15–25m, compared to monotherapy. Similar improvements in exercise capacity have been achieved by exercise and rehabilitation programme in certain patient groups.

Due to a shortage of donor organs, only a minority of suitable patients have heart–lung or lung transplantation which offer a 50% 5-year survival and improved quality of life, but have appreciable morbidity and mortality.

Fundamentally important challenges in the management of PAH include:
- A clear understanding of the biological and molecular mechanisms of the pathogenesis. This should lead to new effective treatments.
- A greater awareness among clinicians that PAH should be investigated as a cause of unexplained breathlessness in a person of any age.
- The development of more accurate non-invasive tests and reliable blood tests for quicker diagnosis and disease management.
- Accurate risk stratification of patients and the identification of those who will benefit most from treatments.
- Evidence from adequately powered, long-term RCTs with clinically relevant endpoints showing that PAH-specific drugs are safe, effective, affordable, and have clinically relevant and beneficial long-term effects.

Due to its enormous diversity encompassing practically all disciplines of medicine, PAH is a condition which is of interest to cardiologists, rheumatologists, chest physicians, haematologists, hepatologists, paediatricians and paediatric cardiologists, transplant surgeons, HIV and infective disease specialists, intensivists, immunologists and inflammation specialists, radiologists, palliative care clinicians, emergency care and general medicine staff, primary care clinicians, hospital managers, and commissioners of treatments and services. This short handbook cannot and does not try to be a PAH textbook covering in depth all the available information and references on PH and PAH. We hope it is helpful to our colleagues as a guide to the current understanding and management of this complex, serious and rapidly changing subject.

Clive Handler

Gerry Coghlan

Acknowledgements

We are grateful to Oxford University Press, the publisher of the *European Heart Journal* for permission to reproduce figures from the 'Guidelines for the diagnosis and treatment of pulmonary hypertension', and Professor Nazzareno Galiè, Chairperson of the The Task Force for the Diagnosis and Treatment of Pulmonary Hypertension of the European Society of Cardiology (ESC) and the European Respiratory Society (ERS), endorsed by the International Society of Heart and Lung Transplantation (ISHLT).

We are also grateful to Professor Dame Carol Black, Professor Christopher Denton, Professor David Abraham, and all our other colleagues working with us in the Centre for Rheumatology and National Pulmonary Hypertension Unit, the Royal Free Hospital, and UCL.

Contents

Detailed contents *xiii*
Symbols and abbreviations *xxi*

Section 1	Pulmonary hypertension in context	1
Section 2	Pathology, pathobiology, and pathophysiology of PAH	23
Section 3	Genetics, epidemiology, and risk factors	59
Section 4	PAH-associated conditions	73
Section 5	Haemodynamics and treatment approaches in PH due to left heart disease	117
Section 6	PH due to chronic lung diseases and/or hypoxia	123
Section 7	Venous thromboembolism, acute pulmonary embolism, and chronic thromboembolic pulmonary hypertension	131
Section 8	Diagnosis and investigations in PAH	153
Section 9	Management of PAH	195

Index *229*

Detailed contents

Symbols and abbreviations *xxi*

Section 1 **Pulmonary hypertension in context**   **1**

1. **History of pulmonary hypertension (PH) and
   the circulation**   **3**
   History of PH and the circulation *4*

2. **Definitions of PH and PAH**   **7**
   PH and PAH *8*
   Normal value of mean pulmonary artery pressure (mPAP) *9*
   Significance of mPAP 21–24mmHg *9*
   mPAP during exercise *9*
   Pulmonary vascular resistance (PVR) *10*
   Pre-capillary versus post-capillary PH *11*
   Post-capillary PH 'out of proportion' to that expected from
     PCWP *14*

3. **The Dana Point (2008) clinical classification of PH**   **15**
   The Dana Point (2008) clinical classification of PH *16*

4. **Prognosis of PAH**   **19**
   Prognosis of PAH *20*

Section 2 **Pathology, pathobiology, and pathophysiology
   of PAH**   **23**

5. **Pathology of PAH**   **25**
   Lung samples *26*
   General pathological findings in PAH *26*

6. **Pathology of pulmonary veno-occlusive disease and
   pulmonary capillary haemangiomatosis**   **29**
   PVOD *30*
   PCH *30*

7. **Pathology of PH due to left heart disease**   31

    Pathology of PH due to left heart disease *32*

8. **Pathology of PH due to lung diseases and/or hypoxia**   33

    Pathology of PH due to lung diseases and/or hypoxia *34*

9. **Pathology of chronic thromboembolic pulmonary hypertension**   35

    Pathology of CTEPH *36*

10. **Pathology of PH with unclear and/or multifactorial mechanisms**   37

    Pathology of PH with unclear and/or multifactorial mechanisms *38*

11. **Pathobiology of PAH**   39

    Pathobiology of PAH *40*

12. **Pathophysiology of PH in non-PAH groups**   41

    Group 2: PH due to left heart disease *42*

    Group 3: PH due to lung diseases and/or hypoxia *42*

    Group 4: CTEPH *43*

13. **Inflammation, growth factors, and thrombosis in PAH**   45

    Inflammation in PAH *46*

    Growth factors and inflammation in PAH *46*

    Cellular factors in PA remodelling *47*

    Viral and other infectious factors in PAH *47*

    Thrombosis in PAH *47*

14. **The pressure loaded right ventricle**   49

    Introduction *50*

    Anatomy *50*

    Pathophysiology *50*

    ECG in right heart disease *52*

    Imaging of the RV *53*

    Invasive assessment of RV *58*

Section 3 **Genetics, epidemiology, and risk factors**   59

15. Genetics and genomics of PAH   61
   Introduction 62
   PAH 62
   Clinical features of HPAH 63
   Genomics in PAH 63
   Genetic testing in PAH 63
   Genetic testing during pregnancy for *BMPR2* mutation carriers 64
   Genetic screening of individuals at risk for PAH 64
   Genetic testing in heritable PAH 64
   Further reading 64

16. Epidemiology of PAH and PH   65
   Introduction 66
   Congenital heart disease-associated PAH 67
   Group 2: PH due to left heart disease 67
   Group 3: Lung diseases with or without hypoxaemia 67
   Group 4: CTEPH 67
   Group 5: PH with unclear and/or multifactorial mechanisms 67
   Prevalence of PAH in subgroups 68

**17. Epidemiology and management of PAH in PVOD
     and/or PCH**   69
   Epidemiology and management of PAH in PVOD
      and/or PCH 70

18. Drugs and toxins and PAH   71
   Introduction 72
   Definite risk factors for PAH 72
   Likely risk factors for PAH 72
   Possible risk factors for PAH 72
   Unlikely risk factors for PAH 72

Section 4 **PAH-associated conditions**   73

19. CTD-associated PAH   75
   Introduction 76
   Systemic sclerosis (scleroderma) 79

Systemic lupus erythematosus *81*

Sjögren's syndrome *86*

Polymyositis and dermatomyositis *86*

20. **PAH associated with HIV**   **87**

Epidemiology of HIV *88*

Virology and immunology *88*

Stages of HIV infection *88*

Management of HIV *89*

HIV and PH *89*

Diagnosis of HIV-PAH *90*

Prognosis *90*

Treatment of HIV-PAH *90*

Further reading *91*

21. **PAH associated with portal hypertension (portopulmonary hypertension)**   **93**

Introduction *94*

Classification of portal hypertension *94*

Pathophysiology of POPH *94*

Screening for POPH *95*

Clinical presentation *95*

Haemodynamics in POPH *95*

Diagnosis of POPH *95*

Medical treatment of POPH *96*

Prognosis of POPH *97*

Further reading *97*

22. **PAH associated with congenital systemic-to-pulmonary cardiac shunts**   **99**

Introduction *100*

Congenital heart disease *100*

Classification of congenital heart disease anomalies associated with PH *101*

Anatomical-pathophysiological classification of congenital systemic-to-pulmonary shunts associated with PAH *102*

Histology of CHD-PAH *104*

Medical treatment for CHD-PAH *104*

Further reading *104*

23. PAH associated with schistosomiasis   105

Introduction *106*

Parasite life cycle *106*

Diagnosis of schistosomiasis *106*

Pathophysiology of schistosomiasis-associated PAH *107*

Chronic schistosomiasis and PAH *107*

Clinical features of schistosomiasis-PAH *107*

Treatment *107*

24. PAH associated with chronic haemolytic anaemias   109

Introduction *110*

Sickle cell disease *110*

Pathophysiology of SCD *110*

Diagnosis of SCD *110*

Sickling crises (painful crisis) and the less common haemolytic,
    sequestration, and aplastic crises *111*

Management of sickle cell crisis *112*

Acute chest crisis *113*

Sickling and NO resistance *113*

Prevalence of PH in SCD *114*

Proposed mechanisms of PAH in SCD *114*

Pathophysiology of PH and PAH in SCD *114*

Long-term management of SCD *114*

Prevention of SCD *115*

Treatment of PAH associated with haemoglobinothies *115*

Section 5 **Haemodynamics and treatment approaches in
         PH due to left heart disease**   **117**

25. Haemodynamics and treatment approaches
in PH due to left heart disease   119

Introduction *120*

Disproportionate post-capillary PH *120*

Presentation of post-capillary PH *120*

Diagnosis of post-capillary PH *121*

Treatment of post-capillary PH *121*

Section 6 **PH due to chronic lung diseases and/or hypoxia** **123**

26. Lung disease-associated PH **125**

Introduction *126*

Diagnostic criteria for IPF (UIP) *127*

Clinical features suggestive of ILD *127*

Histology of IPF *127*

Diagnosing PH in IPF *128*

ILD and SSc-PAH *129*

Treatment of IPF *129*

Treatment of ILD-PH *129*

Classification of ILD *129*

NSIP *130*

Further reading *130*

Section 7 **Venous thromboembolism, acute pulmonary
embolism, and chronic thromboembolic
pulmonary hypertension** **131**

27. Venous thromboembolism **133**

Introduction *134*

Prevalence of VTE *134*

Risk factors for VTE *134*

Pathophysiology and natural history of VTE *135*

Clinical features of DVT *135*

Outcome after VTE and PE *136*

Investigation of VTE and acute PE *136*

Further reading *136*

28. Acute pulmonary embolism and investigations **137**

Clinical features of acute PE *138*

Clinical decision rules *138*

Imaging for suspected acute PE *140*

Treatment of DVT *141*

Treatment of acute PE *142*

Prevention and screening *144*

DVT of the arm *144*

Phlegmasia cerulea dolens *145*

Pregnancy and VTE *145*

Further reading *145*

29. Chronic thromboembolic pulmonary hypertension **147**

Introduction *148*

Anticoagulation *148*

Medical treatment for inoperable CTEPH *148*

Pulmonary endarterectomy *149*

Indications for PEA *150*

Surgical technique *150*

Haemodynamic changes after PEA *150*

Perioperative mortality *150*

Functional class after PEA *150*

Survival in CTEPH *150*

Further reading *151*

Section 8 **Diagnosis and investigations in PAH** **153**

30. Diagnosis and investigations in PAH **155**

General principles of diagnostic approach *156*

Diagnostic algorithm *159*

Simple investigations *161*

V/Q scanning *164*

High resolution computed tomography *166*

Pulmonary angiography and magnetic resonance scanning *167*

Cardiac magnetic resonance imaging (CMR) *171*

Echocardiography *173*

Echocardiographic assessment of the RV *176*

Non-invasive exercise testing *184*

Cardiac catheterization *186*

Acute vasodilator testing *194*

Section 9 **Management of PAH**   **195**

31. **General approach to the management of PAH**   **197**

Introduction *198*

Supportive measures *202*

Contraception in PAH *203*

Risks of pregnancy and contraception *204*

Lifestyle issues *206*

Elective surgery in patients with PAH *207*

Management of arrhythmias *208*

32. **Specific therapies for PAH**   **209**

Supportive medical therapies in PAH *210*

Advanced therapies for PAH *212*

Classes of recommendations for procedures and treatments *218*

Drug interactions with PAH targeted therapies *219*

Combination therapy in PAH *220*

Problems in conducting PAH drug trials *222*

Surgical interventions *225*

Index *229*

Symbols and abbreviations

📖	cross-reference
↑	increased
↓	decreased
~	approximately
±	plus/minus
3D	3-dimensional
ACEi	angiotensin converting enzyme inhibitors
ADD	attention deficit disorder
AF	atrial fibrillation
AIDS	acquired immunodeficiency syndrome
ALK-1	activin-receptor-like kinase
ANA	antinuclear antibody
APAH	associated pulmonary arterial hypertension
APS	antiphospholipid syndrome
AS	atrial septostomy
ASD	atrial septal defect
AV	atrioventricular
AVD	aortic valve disease
BAL	bronchoalveolar lavage
BAS	balloon atrial septostomy
BMPR2	bone morphogenetic protein receptor type 2 gene
BNP	brain natriuretic peptide
BP	blood pressure
bpm	beats per minute
BSA	body surface area
CAD	coronary artery disease
CCB	calcium channel blockers
cGMP	cyclic guanosine monophosphate
CHD	congenital heart disease
CI	cardiac index
CMR	cardiac magnetic resonance
CO	cardiac output
CO_2	carbon dioxide
COPD	chronic obstructive pulmonary disease
CPET	cardiopulmonary exercise testing
CRP	C-reactive protein

CT	computed tomography
CTD	connective tissue disease
CTD-PAH	connective tissue disease-associated pulmonary arterial hypertension
CTED	chronic thromboembolic disease
CTEPH	chronic thromboembolic pulmonary hypertension
CTPA	computed tomography of pulmonary arteries
CTR	cardiothoracic ratio
CXR	chest X-ray
d	day/s
DLCO	diffusion capacity (transfer factor) for carbon monoxide measured on lung function test
ds-DNA	double-stranded deoxyribonucleic acid
DSSc	diffuse systemic sclerosis
DU	duplex ultrasonography
DVT	deep vein thrombosis
EC	endothelial cell
ECG	electrocardiogram
EF	ejection fraction
EMG	electromyography
ENG	endoglin
ERA	endothelin receptor antagonist
ESR	erythrocyte sedimentation rate
ET-1	endothelin-1
FBC	full blood count
FH	family history
GP	general practitioner
GUCH	grown-up congenital heart disease
Hb	haemoglobin
HHT	hereditary haemorrhagic telangiectasia
HIT	heparin-induced thrombocytopenia
HIV	human immunodeficiency virus
HPAH	hereditary pulmonary arterial hypertension
HR	heart rate
HRCT	high resolution computerized tomography of the lungs
IgG	immunoglobulin G
IL	interleukin
ILD	interstitial lung disease
IPAH	idiopathic pulmonary arterial hypertension
IPF	idiopathic pulmonary fibrosis
INR	international normalized ratio

IPF	idiopathic pulmonary fibrosis
IV	intravenous
IVC	inferior vena cava
IVS	interventricular septum
JVP	jugular venous pressure
L	litre/s
LA	left atrium/atrial
LAP	left atrial pressure
LFT	liver function tests
LIVT	liver transplantation
LMWH	low molecular weight heparin
LSSc	limited systemic sclerosis
LT	lung transplantation
LV	left ventricle/ventricular
LVDD	left ventricular diastolic dysfunction
LVEDD	left ventricular end-diastolic diameter
LVEDP	left ventricular end-diastolic pressure
LVESD	left ventricular end-systolic diameter
m	metre/s
MCTD	mixed connective tissue disease
MI	myocardial infarction
min	minute/s
mmHg	mm of mercury
mPAP	mean pulmonary artery pressure
mPCWP	mean pulmonary capillary wedge pressure
MRI	magnetic resonance imaging
MRPA	magnetic resonance pulmonary angiography
MVD	mitral valve disease
NFAT	nuclear factor of activated T cells
NO	nitric oxide
NSAIDs	non-steroidal anti-inflammatory drugs
NSIP	non-specific interstitial pneumonia
NT-proBN	N-terminal fragment of pro-brain natriuretic peptide
O_2	oxygen
PA	pulmonary artery
$PaCO_2$	arterial carbon dioxide tension
PaO_2	arterial oxygen tension
PAH	pulmonary arterial hypertension
PAOP	pulmonary artery occlusion pressure
PAP	pulmonary artery pressure

mPAP	mean pulmonary artery pressure
PASP	pulmonary artery systolic pressure. Estimated PASP = PASP + mRAP
PCH	pulmonary capillary haemangiomatosis
PCWP	pulmonary capillary wedge pressure
PCV	packed cell volume
PDA	patent ductus arteriosus
PDE-5	phosphodiesterase-5
PDE-5I	phosphodiesterase-5 inhibitor
PDGF	platelet-derived growth factor
PE	pulmonary embolism
PEA	pulmonary endarterectomy
PH	pulmonary hypertension
POPH	portopulmonary hypertension
PTS	post-thrombotic syndrome
PVOD	pulmonary veno-occlusive disease
PVR	pulmonary vascular resistance
PWP	pulmonary wedge pressure
RA	right atrium/atrial
RAP	right atrial pressure
RBC	red blood cell
RCT	randomized controlled trial
RFTs	respiratory function test
RHC	right heart catheterization
RhF	rheumatoid factor
RNP	ribonuclear protein
RV	right ventricle/ventricular
RVEDP	right ventricular end-diastolic pressure
RVP	right ventricular pressure
RVSP	right ventricular systolic pressure
s	second/s
6MWT	6 minute walk test
6MWD	6 minute walk distance
SLE	systemic lupus erythematosus
SMC	smooth muscle cell
SSc	systemic sclerosis or scleroderma
SSc-PAH	systemic sclerosis associated pulmonary arterial hypertension
SSRI	selective serotonin reuptake inhibitor
SVC	superior vena cava
SVR	systemic vascular resistance

TAPSE	tricuspid annular plane systolic excursion
TEE	transoesophageal echocardiography
TGF	transforming growth factor signalling family
TLC	total lung capacity
TOE	transoesophageal echocardiography
TPG	transpulmonary pressure gradient (mean PAP − mean PCWP)
TR	tricuspid regurgitation
TTE	transthoracic echocardiography
TV	tricuspid valve
TVR	tricuspid valve regurgitation velocity (m/s). $4 \times TVR^2 =$ PASP
U&E	urea and electrolytes
UFH	unfractionated heparin
UIP	usual interstitial pneumonia
US	ultrasonography
WBC	white blood cell
WHO	World Health Organization
WU	wood units
VC	vital capacity
VCAM-1	vascular cell adhesion molecule-1
VEGF	vascular endothelial growth factor
VIP	vasoactive intestinal polypeptide
V/Q scan	ventilation/perfusion lung scan
VSD	ventricular septal defect
VSMCs	vascular smooth muscle cells
VTE	venous thromboembolism
WHO	World Health Organization
WHO-FC	World Health Organization functional class

Pulmonary hypertension in context

1 History of pulmonary hypertension (PH) and the circulation   **3**

2 Definitions of PH and PAH   **7**

3 The Dana Point (2008) clinical classification of PH   **15**

4 Prognosis of PAH   **19**

History of PH and the circulation

After Harvey's landmark description of the circulation in the mid 17th century, most of the subsequent advances in our understanding of the anatomy and pathophysiology of PH took place in the last century. It is hoped that genetics, molecular biology, translational research, and technical advances will provide further information on this complex condition.

Some of the important contributions are as follows:
- Ibn Nafis 1210–1288: first description of blood flow through the lungs.
- Miguel Serveto 1553: described the pulmonary circulation in his religious treatise *Christianisimi Restitutio*.
- Jacobus Sylvius (1543), Canani (1564), and Fabricius of Aquapendente (1574) concurred in recognizing the centripetal movement of the venous bloodstream from the structure and arrangement of valves in the veins. Before this it had been believed that blood flowed outwards to the periphery, even in the veins.
- Caesalpinus 1569: traced the path of the large circulation.
- William Harvey 1628: *De Motu Cordis et Sanguinis*—first description of the circulation. But he had no clear idea of the circulation in the region of the capillaries.
- Malpighi 1661: described circulation in the capillaries.
- Reverend Stephen Hales 1710: made the first precise measurement of the capacity of a heart. He bled a sheep to death and then led a gun-barrel from the neck vessels into the still-beating heart. Through this, he filled the hollow chambers with molten wax and then measured, from the resultant cast, the volume of the pulse and the cardiac output which he calculated from the pulse rate. Stephen Hales was also the first, in 1727, to record arterial blood pressure, when he measured the rise in a column of blood in a glass tube inserted into an animal's artery.
- William Withering 1785: used digitalis for treatment of oedema and heart failure.
- Chauveau and Marey 1861: measurement of blood pressure inside the heart and the recording of pressure curves from the interior of the heart of a living animal. This was done with manometers, which were led from the neck vessels into both compartments of the right heart and the left heart chamber.
- Adolf Fick 1870: devised a method for measuring cardiac output by dividing oxygen uptake, measured at the mouth, by corresponding arteriovenous difference in oxygen content. The problem of measuring mixed venous oxygen saturation limited the accuracy of his work.
- Ernst von Romberg 1891: first description of pathology of pulmonary arterial hypertension (PAH) in lung arteries, called 'pulmonary vascular sclerosis'.
- Unger, Bleichröder, and Loeb 1912: inserted ureteric catheters, without X-ray visualization, into human patients from the leg arteries up to the presumed height of the bifurcation of the aorta to inject drugs to treat puerperal sepsis. After experiments on animals, they carried out vein experiments on four people as a preliminary trial for intra-arterial therapy. Arrillaga suggested that pulmonary arterial lesions were due to syphilitic endarteritis.

- Montanari 1928: carried out probing of the right heart on animals and on the human cadaver.
- Werner Forssman 1929: self-catheterized his right atrium via his antecubital vein using a ureteral catheter to obtain a mixed venous blood sample.
- Brenner 1935: postmortem study found no evidence that PH was due to syphilis. He described pathology of the small muscular arteries and arterioles.
- Werner Forssman, André Frédéric Cournand, and Dickinson Richards 1956: awarded the Nobel Prize for Medicine.
- HK Hellems and FW Haynes 1950: measurement of pulmonary 'capillary' pressure in humans.
- Dresdale 1951: first clinical diagnosis and further haemodynamic description of 'primary pulmonary hypertension'.
- Paul Wood 1952: demonstrated vasoconstriction of pulmonary arteries in patients with pulmonary hypertension in response to hypoxia.
- M Lategol and H Rahn 1953: use of flow directed catheter to measure pulmonary vascular resistance.
- Heath and Edwards 1958: first histological classification of hypertensive pulmonary vascular disease in patients with congenital heart disease.
- 1960s: aminorex, the appetite suppressant used to aid weight loss, found to be associated with PH. Actions include release of norepinephrine at nerve endings and increase in serotonin levels. Aminorex was withdrawn in 1968. Pulmonary artery lesions at autopsy were identical to lesions found in 'pulmonary arterial hypertension'.
- William Ganz and Harold Swan 1970: multilumen, balloon-tipped catheter to measure pulmonary artery and wedge pressure simultaneously at the bedside, positioned by haemodynamic recording.
- Second epidemic of drug-induced PAH 1990s: dexfenfluramine and phentermine/fenfluramine (phen/fen) led to a 23× ↑ risk of PAH and cardiac valve disease, in drug users compared to age- and gender-matched controls. Both drugs were withdrawn in 1997. Mechanisms of drug-induced PAH remain unclear but are possibly related to a combination of genetic predisposition and the drugs' effects on serotonin uptake.

Definitions of PH and PAH

PH and PAH 8
Normal value of mean pulmonary artery pressure (mPAP) 9
Significance of mPAP 21–24mmHg 9
mPAP during exercise 9
Pulmonary vascular resistance (PVR) 10
Pre-capillary versus post-capillary PH 11
Post-capillary PH 'out of proportion' to that expected
    from PCWP 14

PH and PAH

PH is a haemodynamic and pathophysiological abnormality found in many clinical conditions, most commonly heart and lung diseases.

PH is defined as a mean pulmonary artery pressure (mPAP) of ≥25mmHg (Fig. 2.1).

This is the universally accepted haemodynamic definition published by the European Society of Cardiology,[1] and after the 4th World Symposium on Pulmonary Hypertension.[2]

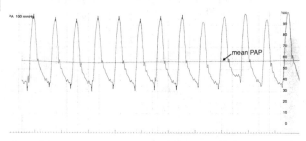

Fig. 2.1 Pulmonary arterial pressure tracing. Scale 0–100mmHg showing a severely elevated mean PAP of 58mmHg. Note the mean pressure line in the middle varies slightly with respiration, and is created as an average of the area under the pressure curve.

Normal value of mean pulmonary artery pressure (mPAP)

The mPAP in healthy individuals is 14±3mmHg with an upper limit of normal of 20mmHg. mPAP during exercise increases with age.

Normal mPAP values
- Normal resting mPAP: 14±3mmHg
- Upper limit of normal: 20mmHg
- mPAP at heart rate of 100bpm: 32mmHg
- Maximal exercise mPAP: 37mmHg
- Exercise in normal person >50 years: 47mmHg.

Significance of mPAP 21–24mmHg

The significance and prognosis of patients with a resting mPAP of 21–24mmHg is unclear. The pulmonary vasculature may not be normal and some individuals with mPAP 21–24mmHg may develop PH. It is not known which individuals progress, why they do, and when this occurs.

mPAP during exercise

Previously, PH was also diagnosed if the mPAP during exercise was ≥30mmHg even if the resting mPAP was <25mmHg.

This is no longer the case because the types and intensity of exercise were not standardized, and the mPAP response to exercise varies with age; healthy individuals commonly exceed a mPAP of 30mmHg during exercise.

Pulmonary vascular resistance (PVR)

PVR is no longer part of the diagnostic criteria for PH or PAH.

$$PVR = \frac{mPAP - mPCWP}{CO}$$

where CO is cardiac output.

Pre-capillary versus post-capillary PH

PH is classified as either pre-capillary PH (PCWP normal and ≤15mmHg) (Fig. 2.2) or post-capillary PH (PCWP elevated and ≥16mmHg) (Table 2.1). This distinction can be made only by cardiac catheterization. RHC is essential for diagnosis and appropriate management.

If the PCWP is unreliable or questionable, the left ventricular end-diastolic pressure (LVEDP) must be obtained by left heart catheterization (Figs. 2.3 and 2.4).

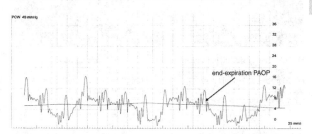

Fig. 2.2 Pulmonary artery occlusion pressure (PAOP) pressure tracing of the same patient as Fig. 2.1. Scale 0–40mmHg. The classical a, c, and v waves are not clearly seen since the a and c waves are hidden within the background 'shatter'. The average line created by the computer is again a running average, because of the much lower pressures and the proportionately greater impact of respiratory pressure changes—the PAOP is recorded as the average pressure at the end of expiration (the point where intrathoracic pressure changes from positive to negative)—7mmHg in this instance.

Table 2.1 Haemodynamic classification of PH

Pre-capillary PH	Post-capillary PH
mPAP ≥25mmHg	mPAP ≥25mmHg
mPCWP ≤15mmHg	PCWP ≥16mmHg
CO normal or reduced	CO normal or reduced
	'Passive' TPG ≤12mmHg
	'Reactive' TPG >12mmHg

TPG, transpulmonary pressure gradient.

Notes: levels recorded at rest, supine.

CO may be reduced by either or both left ventricular impairment (e.g. myocardial infarction [MI], severe aortic valve disease [AVD], mitral regurgitation [MR], myocardial disease), or RV impairment due to severe PH. High CO may be found in systemic to pulmonary shunts, severe anaemia, and hyperthyroidism.

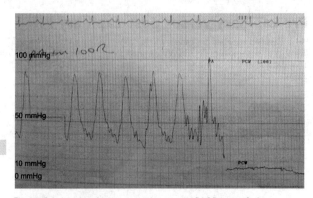

Fig. 2.3 Side-by-side pulmonary arterial tracing and PAOP tracing. Scale 0–100mmHg. The mPAP is 53mmHg, while in this instance a relatively flat looking PAOP tracing at 14mmHg end expiration is obtained. Such presentation is inadequate for diagnostic purposes—since were the true wedge only 2mmHg higher one could not make a diagnosis of PAH.

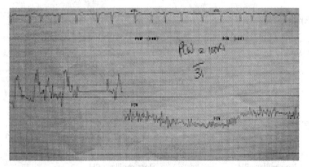

Fig. 2.4 Side-by-side tracings of pulmonary artery and PAOP tracings. Scale 100mmHg. The mPAP is 55mmHg and the end expiration PAOP is 31mmHg. Again, at this scale it is difficult to see if this is a true wedge and further assessments are vital as diagnosis and management are entirely predicated on this PAOP being valid.

Causes of pre-capillary PH

This includes the following groups of PH (groups are numbered according to the clinical classification of PH—see 📖 The Dana Point (2008) clinical classification of PH, p.15):

- 1. PAH
- 3. PH due to lung diseases
- 4. Chronic thromboembolic pulmonary hypertension (CTEPH)
- 5. PH due to unclear or multifactorial mechanisms.

Causes of post-capillary PH

The most common cause of post-capillary PH is left heart disease (systolic and/or diastolic impairment, valvular disease, and constriction) (Fig. 2.5).

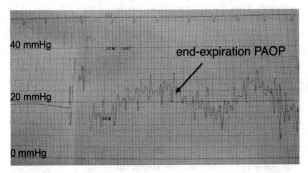

Fig. 2.5 PAOP tracing in a patient with post-capillary pulmonary hypertension. Scale 0–40mmHg. In this particular patient a, c, and v waves are more readily identifiable, improving confidence that this is a true wedge. The end expiration pressure is 24mmHg, and mPAP is always at least 5mmHg higher. Further reassurance can be obtained by assessing the oxygen content of blood aspirated from the wedge position or injecting a small amount of contrast and confirming on fluoroscopy that this does not clear. Identification of the cause of elevation requires assessment of the left ventricular end-diastolic pressure and further investigation of the left heart.

Post-capillary PH 'out of proportion' to that expected from PCWP

The transpulmonary pressure gradient (TPG; mPAP − PCWP) in patients with 'pure' post-capillary PH is 'expected' (defined by current ESC guidelines) to be <12mmHg.

In some patients with post-capillary PH due to left heart disease (valvular disease or left ventricular [LV] impairment), and in chronic obstructive pulmonary disease (COPD), the mPAP is higher than expected; the TPG is >12mmHg and the PVR is >3 Wood units (240 dynes.cms.s−5).

The 'higher than expected' or disproportionately high mPAP may be due to super-added pulmonary vasculopathy due to pulmonary arteriolar vasoconstriction and/or remodelling. The prognostic significance of this observation is not clear. There have been no studies evaluating targeted therapies licensed for this condition, and so there is no evidence that these PAH specific treatments are beneficial.

References

1 Galiè N, Hoeper MM, Humbert M, et al. Guidelines for the diagnosis and treatment of pulmonary hypertension. Eur Heart J 2009; **30**:2493–537.
2 Badesch DB, Champion HC, Sanchez MA, et al. Diagnosis and assessment of pulmonary arterial hypertension. J Am Coll Cardiol 2009; **54**:S55–66.

Further reading

D'Alonzo GE, Barst RJ, Ayres SM, et al. Survival in patients with primary pulmonary hypertension. Results from a national prospective registry. Ann Intern Med 1991; **115**:343–9.
Hatano S, Strasser T (eds). Primary pulmonary hypertension. Geneva: WHO; 1975.
Humbert M, Sitbon O, Chaouat A, et al. Pulmonary arterial hypertension in France: results from a national registry. Am J Respir Crit Care Med 2006; **173**:1023–30.
Kovacs G, Berghold A, Scheidl S, et al. Pulmonary arterial pressure during rest and exercise in healthy subjects. A systematic review. Eur Respir J 2009; **34**(4):888–9.
Oudiz RJ. Pulmonary hypertension associated with left-sided heart disease. Clin Chest Med 2007; **28**:233–41.

The Dana Point (2008) clinical classification of PH

The Dana Point (2008) clinical classification of PH *16*

The Dana Point (2008) clinical classification of PH

PH has been classified into 5 clinical groups according to pathology, pathobiology, genetics, epidemiology, and risk factors.[1]

The prognosis and management of each type of PH depends on the cause or underlying associated condition.

Table 3.1 Classification of PH

1	Pulmonary arterial hypertension (PAH)
1.1	Idiopathic (previously labelled 'primary')
1.2	Heritable (previously labelled 'familial')
1.2.1	*BMPR2*
1.2.2	*ALK-1*, endoglin (with or without hereditary haemorrhagic telangiectasia)
1.2.3	Unknown
1.3	Drugs and toxins induced
1.4	Associated with (APAH)
1.4.1	Connective tissue disease
1.4.2	HIV infection
1.4.3	Portal hypertension
1.4.4	Congenital heart disease
1.4.5	Schistosomiasis
1.4.6	Chronic haemolytic anaemia
1.5	Persistent pulmonary hypertension of the newborn
1'	Pulmonary veno-occlusive disease and/or pulmonary capillary haemangiomatosis
2	Pulmonary hypertension due to left heart disease
2.1	Systolic dysfunction
2.1	Diastolic dysfunction
2.3	Valvular disease
3	Pulmonary hypertension due to lung diseases and/or hypoxia
3.1	Chronic obstructive pulmonary disease
3.2	Interstitial lung disease
3.3	Other pulmonary diseases with mixed restrictive and obstructive pattern
3.4	Sleep-disordered breathing
3.5	Alveolar hypoventilation disorders
3.6	Chronic exposure to high altitude
3.7	Developmental abnormalities
4	Chronic thromboembolic pulmonary hypertension

5	PH with unclear and/or multifactorial mechanisms
5.1	Haematological disorders: myeloproliferative disorders, splenectomy
5.2	Systemic disorders: sarcoidosis, pulmonary Langerhans cell histiocytosis, lymphangioleimyomatosis, neurofibromatosis, vasculitis
5.3	Metabolic disorders: glycogen storage disease, Gaucher disease, thyroid disorders
5.4	Others: tumoural obstruction, fibrosing mediastinitis, chronic renal failure on dialysis

ALK-1, activin receptor-like kinase 1 gene; APAH, associated pulmonary arterial hypertension; *BMPR2*, bone morphogenetic protein receptor, type 2 gene; HIV, human immunodeficiency virus; PAH, pulmonary arterial hypertension.

Reference

1 Simmoneau G, Robbins I, Beghetti M, *et al.* Updated clinical classification of pulmonary hypertension. *J Am Coll Cardiol* 2009; **54**:S43–S54.

Prognosis of PAH

Prognosis of PAH *20*

Prognosis of PAH

- 20 years ago, the median survival of IPAH was 2.8 years.
- Despite earlier and improved detection and the availability of new treatments in the last 10 years, the prognosis with IPAH has improved dramatically with >50% 5 year survival, however the one year mortality remains around 10% in this relatively young population.
- For the 6% of IPAH patients who respond long term to oral CCBs prognosis is excellent with 90% survival at 18 years.
- The natural history of PAH depends on the conditions underlying it. PAH in idiopathic, familial or anorexigen-associated PAH has similar clinical, functional, and haemodynamic characteristics and a similar prognosis.
- The prognosis of PAH-associated with CTD, POPH, and HIV, was worse reflecting the implications of the underlying conditions. However, HIV-associated PAH now has a better survival than IPAH.
- SSc-PAH has a poor prognosis with a survival without treatment of 1 year. The survival is even worse if there is associated, progressive pulmonary fibrosis.

The natural history of PAH is extremely poor. That is why early detection of PAH is important and there is some evidence that the earlier treatment is started the better the outcome.

- Without treatment median survival in class I and II patients is 4.9 years.
- In class III patients is 2.6 years, and
- In class IV patients it is only 6 months (see Fig. 4.1).

Mortality rates are extremely high, comparable to advanced cancer, especially in patients with WHO class III or IV PAH.

Therefore, it is important to treat patients early with therapy that can change the course of disease.

Note: annual screening of patients at high risk for developing PAH (i.e. SSc patients) is recommended in order to be able to initiate early treatment.[1]

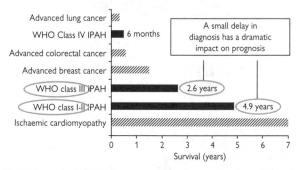

Fig. 4.1 Prognosis of PAH is similar to some advanced cancers. Data from reference 1.

Reference

1 Barst RJ, McGoon M, Torbicki A, *et al.* Diagnosis and differential assessment of pulmonary arterial hypertension. *J Am Coll Cardiol* 2004; **43**:40S–47S.

Further reading

D'Alonzo GE, Barst RJ, Ayres SM, *et al.* Survival in patients with primary pulmonary hypertension. Results from a national prospective registry. *Ann Intern Med* 1991; **115**:343–9.

Section 2

Pathology, pathobiology, and pathophysiology of PAH

5	Pathology of PAH	25
6	Pathology of pulmonary veno-occlusive disease and pulmonary capillary haemangiomatosis	29
7	Pathology of PH due to left heart disease	31
8	Pathology of PH due to lung diseases and/or hypoxia	33
9	Pathology of chronic thromboembolic pulmonary hypertension	35
10	Pathology of PH with unclear and/or multifactorial mechanisms	37
11	Pathobiology of PAH	39
12	Pathophysiology of PH in non-PAH groups	41
13	Inflammation, growth factors, and thrombosis in PAH	45
14	The pressure loaded right ventricle	49

Pathology of PAH

Lung samples 26
General pathological findings in PAH 26

Lung samples

Our understanding of the histology of PAH comes from lungs removed at the time of transplantation and from autopsy. There is very little information from lung tissue removed from a living PAH patient because lung biopsy is dangerous in these sick patients.

General pathological findings in PAH

Fibrotic and proliferative vascular lesions in the small (<500µm in diameter) pulmonary arteries (PAs) are considered responsible for the increase in pulmonary pressures in PAH. The characteristic plexiform lesions vary in frequency.

The distal large and intermediate-sized pulmonary arteries/arterioles are mainly affected with medial and adventitial hypertrophy and hyperplasia, intimal proliferation, concentric and eccentric fibrotic changes, with moderate perivascular inflammatory infiltrates. In advanced cases, complex lesions (plexiform and dilated lesions) are formed from smooth muscle cells, endothelial cells, and fibroblasts), and there is also intravascular thrombosis. Pulmonary veins are not affected. The triggers for these processes are unknown.

Arterial lesions

- Medial hypertrophy, defined as a medial thickness of greater than 10% of the luminal diameter, is seen in all forms of PAH, and in post-capillary PH.
- Medial hypertrophy requires both hypertrophy and smooth muscle hyperplasia, which have been shown to be reversible from studies in patients with high altitude PH.
- Concentric and eccentric non-laminar intimal fibrosis (onion bulb lesions) are common in PAH. These lesions may derive from reactions to damaged endothelium or may develop in response to local thrombosis. Cellular material includes recruited fibroblasts and myofibroblasts. Such lesions are found in all forms of PAH, even where plexiform lesions are uncommon (connective tissue disease-associated PAH [CTD-PAH]). They are strongly associated with plexiform lesions where these are present, suggesting a pattern of histological progression.
- Many other cell types may contribute as staining techniques do not always indicate the origin of cells that become recruited and modified in response to local injury. These lesions are often found in association with plexiform lesions.

Plexiform lesions

- Plexiform lesions were previously thought to be pathognomonic for idiopathic pulmonary arterial hypertension (IPAH), but are also present in portopulmonary hypertension (POPH), CTEPH, and CHD-PH.
- The histological findings are of intimal thickening (Fig. 5.1) followed by exuberant endothelial cell proliferation with sinusoidal channels on a smooth muscle type cell, plus a collagen rich matrix within the native

vessel lumen, obstructing the vessel. These lead into 'dilation' lesions—vein-like structures. Pulmonary haemorrhage in PAH may result from these unstable aneurysmal changes.

- Whether the plexiform lesions represent an attempt to recanalize occluded segments, or lead to shunting is presently unclear. The observation that the endothelial cells within a given lesion are often monoclonal, raises the possibility of a neoplastic-like response to injury at these sites.

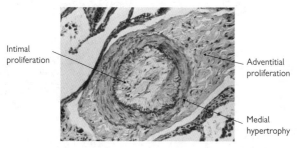

Intimal proliferation

Adventitial proliferation

Medial hypertrophy

Fig. 5.1 (Also see Colour plate 1.) A plexiform lesion in a small pulmonary arteriole showing intimal and medial disruption and hypertrophy, aneurysmal dilatation, and formation of a complex proliferative tuft of intimal cells and channels. Published with permission from S Gaine and L Rubin.

Vasculitic lesions

Vasculitic lesions are rare in PAH—these are characterized by transmural inflammation and fibrinoid necrosis. However, perivascular inflammatory cell infiltrates are not uncommon in PAH, especially in association with plexiform lesions.

Venous lesions

- Loose fibrous remodelling of the intima may be found in both the septal veins and preseptal venules. Abnormalities of the septal veins occur in a number of conditions associated with ↑ post-capillary pressure and alone, are not considered diagnostic of PAH. Diagnosis depends on the site of the dominant histological abnormality since patients with PAH may have some changes in the pulmonary veins and patients with PVOD may have some changes in the PAs.
- Changes in septal veins comprise loose paucicellular fibrous obstruction.
- Preseptal venules often present dense fibrous occlusion often with ↑ cellularity. Smooth muscle cells or myofibroblasts are often evident within such lesions, and thrombotic material may be evident. ↑ muscularization of the venules may be present.
- Significant haemosiderin deposits are frequently found in association with PVOD, suggesting that subclinical pulmonary haemorrhage is common.

Further reading

Pietra GG, Capron F, Stewart S, et al. Pathologic assessment of vasculopathies in pulmonary hypertension. *J Am Coll Cardiol* 2004; **43**:S25–S32.

Tuder RM, Abman SH, Braun T, et al. Development and pathology of pulmonary hypertension. *J Am Coll Cardiol* 2009; **54**:S3–S9.

Pathology of pulmonary veno-occlusive disease and pulmonary capillary haemangiomatosis

PVOD *30*
PCH *30*

PVOD

- PVOD is a rare pulmonary vascular disease causing PH. The incidence is 0.1–0.2 per million per year. The preseptal and septal venules are affected and become fibrotic and thickened due to cellular proliferation.
- The characteristic findings are: occlusive fibrotic lesions, venous muscularization, patchy capillary proliferation, pulmonary oedema, lymphatic dilatation, lymph node enlargement, and inflammatory infiltrates. Occult pulmonary haemorrhage is common in PVOD probably due to post-capillary block.
- Medial hypertrophy, intimal fibrosis, and complex lesions affect the distal pulmonary PAs.

PCH

- PCH is a rare condition associated with progressive dyspnoea and pulmonary haemorrhage. Histologically there is aggressive alveolar septal capillary proliferation and thickening. Occult haemorrhage or haemosiderosis is common.
- Diffuse perivenular foci of capillary proliferation occur in both PCH and PVOD.

Pathology of PH due to left heart disease

Pathology of PH due to left heart disease *32*

Pathology of PH due to left heart disease

- The pulmonary veins are enlarged and thickened and the pulmonary capillaries are dilated.
- There is interstitial oedema, alveolar haemorrhage, lymphatic vessel, and lymph node enlargement.
- There may be medial hypertrophy and intimal fibrosis of the distal PAs.

Pathology of PH due to lung diseases and/or hypoxia

Pathology of PH due to lung diseases and/or hypoxia *34*

Pathology of PH due to lung diseases and/or hypoxia

- Medial hypertrophy and intimal obstructive proliferation of the distal PAs. In emphysema and lung fibrosis, the vascular bed is affected.
- In advanced lung disease, the loss of capillary cross-sectional area is believed to be responsible for PH, although this has not been confirmed on histological evaluation, and there is a very poor relationship between the extent of lung destruction and the severity of PH. While there have been some observations of medial thickening as in PAH, this is generally quite mild, hence there is no rational basis for treating these patients with PAH therapies.
- In hypoxaemia, hypoxic-inducible factor promotes vasospasm and medial proliferation. Although vasodilators and antiproliferative therapies may, theoretically, have a role, there is no clinical evidence for this. Oxygen is the most important treatment and reduces pulmonary pressures.

Pathology of chronic thromboembolic pulmonary hypertension

Pathology of CTEPH 36

Pathology of CTEPH

- CTEPH results from obstruction of the pulmonary arterial bed by non-resolving thromboemboli, and fibrous stenosis and/or complete obliteration of the PA. Acute pulmonary emboli (PEs) are probably the initiating event. Most patients with acute PEs recover spontaneously. The minority who do not, develop progressive pulmonary occlusions and a generalized hypertensive pulmonary arteriopathy with remodelling of the smaller vessels not affected by the thrombosis. This scenario would explain why some patients have severe PH despite what appears to be mild pulmonary vascular thrombosis. There are often associated distal thromboemboli in subsegmental vessels and are thus inaccessible from an operative standpoint.
- Organized thrombi attached to the medial layer of the pulmonary arteries, and are covered on the luminal side by neointima. These lesions may completely obstruct the lumen or form webs, stenoses, or bands in the PAs. Histologically the material retrieved is fibroelastic subendothelial obstruction, rather than thrombus.
- In the non-occluded areas of the lungs, a pulmonary arteriopathy indistinguishable from that of PAH can develop. There may be collaterals to the PAs from the systemic circulation (bronchial, costal, diaphragmatic, and coronary arteries) which partially reperfuse areas distal to the complete obstructions.

Further reading

Fedullo PF, Auger WR, Kerr KM, et al. Chronic thromboembolic pulmonary hypertension. *N Engl J Med* 2001; **345**:1465–72.

Pathology of PH with unclear and/ or multifactorial mechanisms

Pathology of PH with unclear and/or multifactorial
   mechanisms 38

Pathology of PH with unclear and/or multifactorial mechanisms

There are no characteristic pathological features for this heterogeneous group.

Pathobiology of PAH

Pathobiology of PAH 40

Pathobiology of PAH

The cause of PAH remains unclear. Several mechanisms have been proposed, involving multiple biochemical pathways and cell types.

Endothelial dysfunction leads to an increase in PVR via several mechanisms:
- Vasoconstriction due to chronically impaired production of vasodilator and antiproliferative agents such as nitric oxide (NO), vasoactive intestinal polypeptide (VIP), and prostacyclin, along with overexpression of vasoconstrictor and proliferative substances such as thromboxane A_2 and endothelin. VIP, a vasodilator, and antiproliferative levels are reduced.
- Proliferation of the walls of the PAs leading to luminal obstruction with apoptosis resistant cells.
- Inflammation.
- Thrombosis.
- Abnormal function and expression of potassium channels in the vascular smooth muscle cells (VSMCs).

These abnormalities are mediated in part by a reduced production of prostacyclin, NO, and overexpression of endothelin. These are the targets for current drug treatment of PAH.
- Prostacyclin is a potent vasodilator of all vascular beds. It is antiproliferative, a potent inhibitor of platelet aggregation, and is cytoprotective.
- Prostacyclin and synthetic prostanoids were the first effective treatments for PAH and remain important drugs.
- NO production is reduced. NO is a powerful vasodilator and antiproliferative substance. Phosphodiesterase-5 (PDE-5) breaks down NO. This is the rationale for PDE-5 inhibitors in treating PAH—they produce vasodilatation and exert antiproliferative effects.
- Overexpression of vasoconstrictor and proliferative substances e.g. thromboxane A2 and endothelin-1. This is the rationale for endothelin receptor antagonists (ERA) in treating PAH.
- Other vasodilator and antiproliferative substances, e.g. VIP, are also reduced.
- These changes induce remodelling and thickening of the PA walls by proliferation, vasoconstriction, fibrosis by VSMCs, endothelial cells, and fibroblasts.

The adventitia

In the adventitia there is ↑ production of extracellular matrix including collagen, elastin, fibronectin, tenascin, and matrix-bound smooth muscle cell mitogens, such as basic fibroblast growth factor. Other matrix metalloproteases can stimulate the production of tenascin, a smooth muscle cell mitogenic cofactor.

Further reading

Hassoun PM, Mouthon L, Barbera JA, et al. Inflammation, growth factors, and pulmonary vascular remodeling. *J Am Coll Cardiol* 2009; **54**:S10–S19.

Humbert M, Morrell NW, Archer SL, et al. Cellular and molecular pathobiology of pulmonary arterial hypertension. *J Am Coll Cardiol* 2004; **43**:S13–S24.

Morrell N, Adnot S, Archer S, et al. Cellular and molecular basis of pulmonary arterial hypertension. *J Am Coll Cardiol* 2009; **54**:S20–S31.

Pathophysiology of PH in non-PAH groups

Group 2: PH due to left heart disease 42
Group 3: PH due to lung diseases and/or hypoxia 42
Group 4: CTEPH 43

Group 2: PH due to left heart disease

PH is common in all forms of left heart disease. Any cause of an increase in LVEDP (coronary heart disease, cardiomyopathy, valvular heart disease) results in an increase in LAP, which is transmitted by passive back pressure through the pulmonary veins to the PA (post-capillary PH). The TPG should be <12mmHg. The PVR is usually normal.

- If the TPG is abnormally high because the increase in mPAP is greater than the increase in PCWP, and the PVR is also abnormally high, this is called post-capillary reactive or 'out-of-proportion' PH.
- This increase in PVR may be due to ↑ vasomotor tone of the PAs and/ or fixed obstruction of the PAs due to remodelling of the PAs with intimal proliferation and medial hypertrophy. This causes narrowing of PAs and arterioles.
- The increase in vasomotor tone may respond to vasodilators during a vasodilator challenge or with drugs. Fixed obstruction would not respond to a vasodilator challenge.
- The mechanisms of these processes are not well understood, however abnormal endothelial function has been reported, including ↑ endothelin production and reduced NO and PG production.

Group 3: PH due to lung diseases and/ or hypoxia

The pathophysiology of PH in this group is incompletely understood. Hypoxia is the main cause of PH. Where lung disease is advanced, there is no role for specific therapy for PAH. In many patients a judgement must be made whether a modest reduction in lung function is sufficient to explain the degree of PH observed.

Pulmonary function testing is helpful in patients with elevated pulmonary pressures. Substantial reductions in lung volumes (FVC or TLC <70% predicted) or FEV$_1$/FVC <60% indicate significant lung disease. Reductions in gas transfer are more difficult to interpret as these can be reduced in pulmonary vascular disease, especially in the setting of CTD and in smokers.

Group 4: CTEPH

Although hereditary thrombophilia is associated with DVTs and venous thromboembolism (VTE), this association does not exist with CTEPH where PEs do not resolve and obstruct PAs increasing PAP. It is not clear to what extent the pulmonary vasculature has to be obstructed to cause PH. The histology of the lesions in CTEPH are similar to those found in PAH and may be due to shear stress, pressure, inflammation, and the release of cytokines and vasculotrophic mediators.

Hereditary thrombophilia and *in situ* thrombosis is found only occasionally in CTEPH. 10% of patients have lupus anticoagulant, 20% have antiphospholipid antibodies, lupus anticoagulant, or both and 40% have raised factor VIII protein which is associated with primary and recurrent VTE.

Splenectomy, thrombophilia, ventriculo-atrial shunt for the treatment of hydrocephalus, osteomyelitis, central venous cannulas which have been inserted for more than a few months, myeloproliferative disorders, and chronic inflammatory bowel diseases, increase the risk of CTEPH. The causes for this ↑ risk are not clear.

Given the lack of association with abnormalities that cause excessive coagulation or fibrinolysis, it is presently postulated that abnormal thrombus organization leads to fibrous transformation of clot observed in CTEPH.

Inflammation, growth factors, and thrombosis in PAH

Inflammation in PAH 46
Growth factors and inflammation in PAH 46
Cellular factors in PA remodelling 47
Viral and other infectious factors in PAH 47
Thrombosis in PAH 47

Inflammation in PAH

- Inflammation plays a role in IPAH and CTD-PAH, HIV-PAH, with circulating antinuclear antibody (ANA) and ↑ levels of pro-inflammatory cytokines interleukin (IL)-1 and IL-6. Inflammatory cells and platelets through the serotonin pathway may play a role.
- Inflammatory cells: macrophages, T and B lymphocytes, and dendritic cells are present in plexiform vascular lesions in IPAH, CTD-PAH, HIV-PAH. Macrophage inflammatory proteins are ↑ in severe PAH.
- Circulating chemokines and cytokines, viral protein components, and ↑ expression of growth (e.g. vascular endothelial growth factor [VEGF], platelet-derived growth factor [PDGF]) and transcriptional (e.g. nuclear factor of activated T cells [NFAT]) factors are believed to contribute directly to further recruitment of inflammatory cells, proliferation of smooth muscle cells (SMCs) and endothelial cells.
- These inflammatory disturbances offer potential specific targets for new therapies.

Growth factors and inflammation in PAH

The growth factors, epidermal growth factor (EGF), VEGF, and PDGF are implicated in abnormal proliferation and migration of PA vascular cells. These growth factors are potent mitogens and chemoattractants for SMCs, fibroblasts, and endothelial cells (ECs) and cause resistance to apoptosis. All have been reported to be ↑ (the molecule and/or the specific receptors) in the lung and/or in the blood of PAH patients.

- *VEGF* is a mediator of angiogenesis but also a factor involved in permeability and inflammatory processes in the vascular endothelium.
- *PDGF* is synthesized by many different cell types including SMCs, ECs, and macrophages. PDGF induces proliferation and migration of SMCs and fibroblasts and is implicated in several fibroproliferative disorders, including PAH. PDGF is overproduced and promotes remodelling in PAH.
- *EGF* is implicated in proliferation and migration of SMCs in PAH and is dependent on the extracellular matrix component, tenascin C.
- *Serotonin (5-HT) and serotonin transporter (5-HTT):* 5-HT is mitogenic and constricts PA-SMCs via 5-HTT. Drugs that inhibit 5-HTT block the mitogenic effects of 5-HT on SMCs.
  - 5-HT levels are ↑ in PAH.
  - 5-HTT is located in PA-SMCs, and is involved in PA remodelling. Transgenic mice with selective overexpression of 5-HT in SMCs spontaneously develop PAH. These effects are blocked by 5-HTT blockers.
  - 5-HTT is ↑ in platelets and the media of thickened PAs in IPAH. 5-HTT overexpression in PA-SMCs in IPAH patients may increase mitogenic response to 5-HT.

- PA-SMC hyperplasia in IPAH appears to result from both dysregulation of 5-HT production by ECs due to overexpression of tryptophan hydroxylase-1 and from ↑ PA-SMC response to 5-HT due to expression of 5-HTT.
- *Survivin and PA vascular remodelling:* survivin is an inhibitor of apoptosis. Dysregulation of survivin is linked to malignant processes. Survivin is overexpressed in PAs from PAH patients and in rats with MCT-induced PAH.
  - Gene therapy with an adenovirus carrying a mutant form of survivin reverses MCT-PAH and prolongs survival and improves haemodynamics.
  - *In vitro*, inhibition of endogenous survivin induces PA-SMC apoptosis.
  - The normal absence of survivin in healthy tissues suggests it is a potential target for therapy.

Cellular factors in PA remodelling

Mitochondrial and ion channel dysregulation appear to convey cellular resistance to apoptosis and vascular wall hypertrophy.

Viral and other infectious factors in PAH

- Several infectious agents have been suggested to play a role in PAH including Epstein–Barr virus, hepatitis C, and HIV, where the prevalence of PAH is 0.46% vs 0.0002% in the general population. HIV-PAH is independent of CD4+ T-cell counts and antiviral drug treatment.
- Very little is known about the molecular mechanisms that are responsible for virus-related PH.

Thrombosis in PAH

Prothrombotic abnormalities have been demonstrated in PAH and thrombi are present in the small distal PAs and the proximal elastic PAs.

Chapter 14

The pressure loaded right ventricle

Introduction 50
Anatomy 50
Pathophysiology 50
ECG in right heart disease 52
Imaging of the RV 53
Invasive assessment of RV 58

Introduction

Prognosis and symptoms in PAH are determined largely by RV function. Compared to the LV, the RV is difficult to image and evaluate haemodynamically because of its anatomy and interrelationship with the LV, its geometry, and its sensitivity to alterations in pulmonary pressure. It also fails comparatively early in response to pressure overload.

Anatomy

The RV is located immediately behind the sternum, is triangular and wraps, around the LV. The RV wall is 3–5mm thick. Contraction relies more on longitudinal shortening rather than circumferential shortening. It is divided into 3 anatomical and functional components:

- Inlet portion from tricuspid valve to insertion of papillary muscles on to the ventricular walls.
- Trabecular portion involving the RV body and apex (the main part of the pump).
- Outflow or infundibular portion extending to the pulmonary valve.

The RV is difficult to image with echocardiography because of its triangular shape and trabeculated and crescentic cavity which make internal measurements very difficult.

With pressure overload and hypertrophy, the RV wall may exceed the thickness of the LV.

Pathophysiology

The RV is more compliant than the LV. It adapts to volume loading but not to prolonged pressure loading. Physiologically, it is connected to the low-pressure pulmonary circulation. The shared interventricular septum means that any impairment of either chamber affects the other (ventricular interdependence) (Fig. 14.1).

- ↑ RVEDP leads to systolic flattening of the IVS which may bulge into the LV when RVP increases to high levels. This results in impaired LV filling and contraction. In acute PE, the RV dilates with hypokinesia of the free wall.
- In PAH, the RV wall is affected by similar pathological processes as the PAs, with hypertrophy, fibrosis, inflammation, myocyte apoptosis and necrosis, and global impaired function.
- As RV function deteriorates and the RV dilates due to increases in RVEDP, the TV annulus is stretched causing TR, leading to further deterioration in forward flow to the lungs.
- Early filling of the RV is reduced as RVEDP increases, leading to reversal of the transtricuspid E:A ratio, which may then pseudonormalize as the RAP increases.
- The myocardial vascular response to hypertrophy is not fully matched, and with increasing RV systolic pressure systolic coronary flow to the RV is lost leading to myocardial ischaemia and angina in severe PH.

- Although RV failure clearly results from unrelieved PAH and is the dominant cause of death, it is not clear that this is due to myocyte damage as seen in LV failure, since the RV will recover with offloading as seen in CTEPH surgery, post LT and in those who normalize pressures on vasodilator therapy.

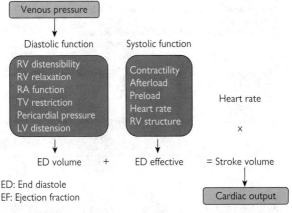

Fig. 14.1 Factors affecting RV performance. Cardiac index and right atrial pressure are the most important haemodynamic measurements when estimating prognosis in pulmonary hypertension. The diagram shows that these measurements are dependent not just on RV myocyte contractile function and loading conditions but also RV geometry, diastolic function and LV shape and size all of which are affected in PH.

ECG in right heart disease

The following features may be seen in isolation or various combinations in severe PH and/or right heart failure (Fig. 14.2):

- Tachycardia.
- Right-axis deviation.
- Dominant R wave V1 (only 1 of 6 causes).
- Big P waves (P pulmonale—more than 2mV in lead II).
- Right bundle branch block.
- ST–T wave changes in V1–V3 and the inferior leads.

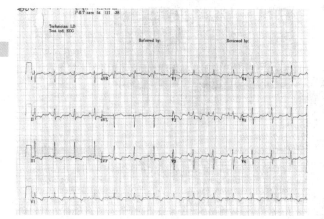

Fig. 14.2 Typical ECG in pulmonary hypertension: right axis deviation (leads I and aVL are dominantly negative, while lead II is positive), RV hypertrophy (dominant R wave in V1 with an rsR' pattern and an S wave in V6) and RV strain (ST depression and T wave inversion V2–V4 and in some cases extending to the inferior leads as shown here).

Imaging of the RV

CXR

This is unreliable in sizing the RV because of the configuration of the RV. The CTR may be normal even if the RV is enlarged because of compression of the LV (Fig. 14.3).

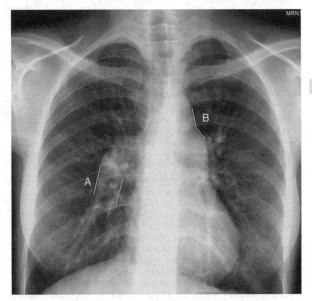

Fig. 14.3 Chest radiograph of a patient with PAH. Note gross enlargement of the PAs such that the right PA is grossly enlarged (A: normal <16mm) and the angle between the aortic knuckle and the left PA is lost (B: normal <90°). Despite these gross changes the cardiothoracic ratio remains below 0.5.

Echocardiography

- Evaluating RV function by measuring RV volume is complicated because contractility is highly dependent on filling pressures (preload), pulmonary pressures (afterload), HR (force frequency relationship), and RV shape and size which changes as pressures rise; further the RV geometry complicates simple measurements.
- Load-independent measures such as the TEI index (non-ejecting contraction time relative to total contraction time) and TAPSE (a simple measure of longitudinal function) attempt to overcome the difficulties of measuring RV function.
- Echocardiography will show evidence of RV pressure and volume overload except in early PH.
- RA area enlargement, RV end-diastolic internal diameter ≥LV internal diameter at end diastole just below AV valve insertion, distortion of the LV from its normal circular appearance in short-axis views, and pericardial effusion due to heart failure are among the most reliable features.

Although echocardiography has limitations in measuring RV function, it is most helpful when the RV is dilated in advanced PAH. Gross dilatation of the RV with compression of the LV is a clear sign of pressure overload. RA dilation is a very consistent sign of adverse prognosis, as this provides indirect evidence of reduced RV diastolic or systolic function (Figs. 14.4 and 14.5).

Developing methods may overcome some of the limitations of echocardiographic assessment.

- Strain and strain-rate assessments allow real-time assessment of the regional degree of contraction in the RV.
- These techniques are limited by the very thin wall of the normal RV and the difficulty obtaining high-quality images of the myocardium at high frame rates such that the speckles tracked in deriving such information may not be reproducible.
- Vector velocity imaging combines feature tracking, endocardial tracking, speckle tracking, and RR periodicity to provide comprehensive directional and velocity assessment of all imaged sections of the RV throughout the cardiac cycle. Though only presently possible in 2 dimensions this may improve understanding of the changes in RV function over time.
- Through ESPVR assessment (end systolic pressure volume relationships) using tricuspid velocity to assess end systolic pressure and 3-dimensional (3D) echo to assess volume we may get closer to using this measure that has proven important in understanding LV function in heart failure.

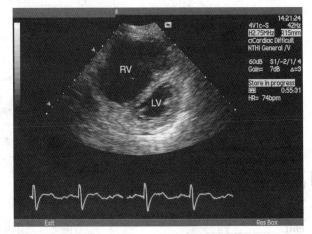

Fig. 14.4 Septal flattening: short-axis view on echocardiography showing an enlarged right ventricular cavity in the upper left of the picture (RV) and a compressed left ventricular cavity in the lower right of the picture (LV). The septum which separates these is flattened distorting the usually circular outline of the LV cavity in this view.

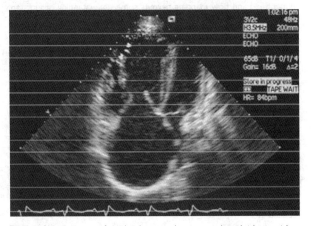

Fig. 14.5 LV compression: four-chamber view showing an enlarged right ventricle (RV) and right atrium (RA) compressing the left ventricle (LV) and atrium (LA). Normally in this view the left heart dominates the right.

Left heart disease and PH

- In severe PH, the enlarged RV causes deviation of the interventricular septum (IVS) and compression of the LV. Standard measures may suggest reduced LV function.
- PH may also be due to LV impairment and dilatation. Signs of MI with regional wall movement abnormalities and thinning of the LV due to infarction may be present.
- Echocardiographic features include: increases in LVEDD to >5.9cm, LVESD to >4.0cm. Systemic hypertension may cause post-capillary PH. Echocardiographic features include: LV hypertrophy with increases in the IVS >1.1cm, posterior LV wall to >1.1cm, and the LA diameter to >4.5cm or LA area > 18cm^2. Both left heart systolic and diastolic dysfunction may cause PH.
- Signs of restriction and constriction, valve abnormalities, and shunts or other evidence of CHD should be excluded.

Where echocardiography suggests a left heart cause for PH, catheterization with coronary angiography may be appropriate and provides further useful diagnostic information.

MRI

The limitations of echocardiography are largely overcome by the use of cardiac magnetic resonance imaging, the resolution is much greater, the location of the RV does not affect image quality and 3D reconstruction is readily achieved (Fig. 14.6). In addition, use of gadolinium enhancement allows areas of replacement fibrosis in response to myocardial damage to be identified and flow mapping permits some understanding of function. MRI therefore permits:

- Volumetric assessment of the entire RV in systole and diastole.
- Assessment of RV mass and change over time.
- Assessment of flow pattern in the PAs.
- Assessment of tricuspid regurgitation.
- Analysis of cardiac and associated vascular structures—identifying congenital abnormalities and vascular obstructions.
- Assessment of fibrosis or myocardial inflammation.
- Tagged imaging permits assessment of strain and strain rate assessment of the myocardium throughout the RV throughout contraction and relaxation.

MRI is therefore a very powerful tool, but limitations exist—it is as yet not commonly available, assessment of end-systolic volume and shape is hampered by the size and location of trabeculae, assessments of mass are non-standardized as there is disagreement about how to manage the RV septal contribution to mass, flow assessments tend to suggest different stroke volumes from the left and right ventricles and are therefore not yet accurate.

Without the ability to measure real-time pressures, this technique cannot give insights into the pressure volume relationships in the RV, therefore understanding of the contractile function of the RV remains limited.

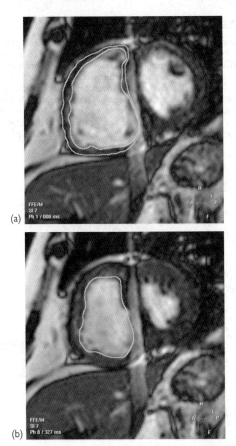

Fig. 14.6 Short axis MRI tomogram of the heart. Figure (a): the diastolic image of the right ventricle (RV). Figure (b): the systolic image of the right ventricle. In figure (a), the outer white line traces the epicardial border of the RV, and the inner white line, the endocardial border of the RV. The septum is flattened and assumed to contribute at least 50% of its mass to the RV. The difference between these areas can be used to calculate RV mass area and through summation from multiple slices, myocardial volume. Assuming the density of myocardium is constant, the RV mass can be assessed. In figure (b), the white line traces the end-systolic area; again, through summation of multiple slices, the difference between the end-diastolic and end-systolic volumes can be measured and used to estimate ventricular ejection fraction.

Invasive assessment of RV

Simultaneous, real-time pressure and volume measurements of the RV are required. The rapid changes in pressure in the RV means that standard fluid-filled catheters (inaccurate above 10–12Hz) do not provide real-time pressure information, and volume assessments are limited to stroke volume. These limitations are partly overcome by using solid state pressure transducers and volumetric assessments using conductance catheters, but even with such advanced technology, the shape of the RV limits the accuracy of volume assessments. Until invasive and MRI volume assessments are undertaken simultaneously, our understanding of the RV is limited.

Genetics, epidemiology, and risk factors

15	Genetics and genomics of PAH	**61**
16	Epidemiology of PAH and PH	**65**
17	Epidemiology and management of PAH in PVOD and/or PCH	**69**
18	Drugs and toxins and PAH	**71**

Chapter 15

Genetics and genomics of PAH

Introduction 62
PAH 62
Clinical features of HPAH 63
Genomics in PAH 63
Genetic testing in PAH 63
Genetic testing during pregnancy for *BMPR2*
    mutation carriers 64
Genetic screening of individuals at risk for PAH 64
Genetic testing in heritable PAH 64
Further reading 64

Introduction

- PAH may be hereditable (formerly termed 'familial').
- One aetiological theory for PAH is an interaction between bone morphogenetic protein receptor type 2 (*BMPR2*) disease mutations and environmental exposures (e.g. viral infection, anorexigenic drugs, some hormones). Genetic mutations are, however, neither necessary nor sufficient to cause PAH.
- All case/control analyses of IPAH suffer from critically small sample cohorts and the crucial 2nd stage of association analyses are often lacking in genetic studies.
- It is now possible to analyse several hundred thousand independent loci and this may improve our understanding of the human heliotypic architecture of sequence variation and identification of loci conferring even modest risks for PAH. This, however, requires large numbers of cases and controls.

PAH

Idiopathic PAH corresponds to sporadic disease in which there is neither a family history (FH) of PAH nor an identified risk factor. When PAH occurs in a familial context, germline mutations in the *BMPR2* gene, a member of the TGFβ signalling family, can be detected in >70% of cases of HPAH.

- As in other similar genetic conditions, parents may feel guilty to find that they have passed on a mutation to their child.
- In 2000, *BMPR2* was identified following linkage analysis. Nearly 300 *BMPR2* mutations have been identified.
- Crude indirect estimates of the population carrier frequency for *BMPR2* mutations lie in the range of 0.001–0.01%. More rarely, mutations in activin receptor-like kinase type 1 (*ALK1*), or endoglin (*ENG*), also members of the TGFβ signalling family, have been identified in PAH patients, commonly with coexistent hereditary haemorrhagic telangiectasia (HHT).
- *BMPR2* mutations are found in 11–40% of apparently idiopathic cases of PAH with no family history. The distinction between idiopathic and familial *BMPR2* genes is artificial. All patients with *BMPR2* mutations have heritable disease. Therefore, around 20% of patients with IPAH have mutations in *BMPR2* and the potential risk to family members should be considered. A FH of PAH may not be recognized in IPAH cases with *BMPR2* mutations because of incomplete penetrance, absence of phenotyic consequences, or new spontaneous mutations.
- HPAH is inherited as an autosomal dominant trait with incomplete penetrance. Lifetime penetrance is only 10–20% and there are no known preventative measures.
- ♀:♂ = 1.7:1.
- Heritable forms of PAH include sporadic cases of IPAH with germline mutations (mainly *BMPR2* but also *ALK1* or *ENG*) and familial cases with or without identified germline mutations.

Clinical features of HPAH

- HPAH and IPAH have similar clinical features. PAH patients with *BMPR2* mutations are less likely to respond to acute vasodilator testing or calcium channel blockers.
- PAH may be associated with HHT (also known as Osler–Weber–Rendu syndrome) in which vascular lesions are a characteristic feature, and mutations in the *ALK1* gene are present.

Genomics in PAH

With international collaboration, genome-wide association studies will be conducted to identify additional genes for HPAH, genetic modifiers for BMPR2 penetrance, and genetic susceptibility to IPAH.

Genetic testing in PAH

- Clinical genetic testing is available for PAH for *BMPR2*, *ALK1*, and *ENG*. The most common requests from parents for genetic testing are to see if children have a hereditary predisposition to PAH or to make informed choices about family planning.
- In the USA the Genetics Information Nondiscrimination Act 2008 protects members of both individual and group insurance plans from discrimination in coverage or health insurance coverage and also protects against discrimination in employment based upon genetic predisposition.
- Routine genetic testing is not necessary in all IPAH or in familial PAH. Genetic testing is appropriate as part of a comprehensive programme including genetic counselling, and discussions of the risks and benefits and limitations of such testing.
- Genetic testing in children raises ethical issues and should be performed with caution because of the potentially significant psychological impact on the child learning that they may develop a potentially fatal disease without a known cure.
- Identification of a familial mutation can be valuable in reproductive planning and identifying family members who are not mutation carriers and so will not need lifelong surveillance.
- Molecular genetic testing may be indicated in familial PAH following comprehensive genetic counselling for resolution of individual risk and family planning. Joint care between the PAH centre and the genetic centre is advised.

Genetic testing during pregnancy for *BMPR2* mutation carriers

- There is a 50% risk of transmitting a *BMPR2* mutation from mother to fetus.
- Prenatal testing of a fetus for *BMPR2* mutations in carriers of this mutation is available using chorionic villus sampling in the 10th week of pregnancy. This is not commonly requested because of the reduced penetrance of PAH mutations.
- Another approach is pre-implantation genetic diagnosis. Families use *in vitro* fertilization of a tested embryo, free of the *BMPR2* mutation, prior to implantation.

Genetic screening of individuals at risk for PAH

This is controversial because, as in other situations, e.g. CTD-PAH, there is little evidence that early diagnosis and treatment improves outcomes. However, studies in patients with HPAH and carriers of *BMPR2* mutations are in progress with non-invasive screening using clinical examination, Doppler echocardiography, and stress echocardiography and stress testing. A recommendation without much evidence to support it is that relatives should be screened, 'periodically'.

Genetic testing in heritable PAH

- The indications for clinical and genetic screening in IPAH are unclear. It appears that 1st- and 2nd-degree relatives of patients with IPAH are at low risk. Parents of children with PAH should be counselled about the potential risks, benefits, and limitations of genetic testing for future pregnancies and siblings. The recurrence rate for siblings is low and estimated at <5%. The age of onset of IPAH may vary within families.
- The genetics of associated forms of PAH are unclear.
- Recognized familial cases of IPAH should be offered family-based risk assessment and genetic counselling.

Further reading

Machado RD, Aldred MA, James V, *et al.* Mutations of the TGF-beta type II receptor BMPR2 in pulmonary arterial hypertension. *Hum Mutat* 2006; **27**:121–32.

Machado R, Eickelberg O, Elliott CG, *et al.* Genetics and genomics of pulmonary arterial hypertension. *J Am Coll Cardiol* 2009; **54**:S32–42.

Epidemiology of PAH and PH

Introduction 66
Congenital heart disease-associated PAH 67
Group 2: PH due to left heart disease 67
Group 3: Lung diseases with or without hypoxaemia 67
Group 4: CTEPH 67
Group 5: PH with unclear and/or multifactorial mechanisms 67
Prevalence of PAH in subgroups 68

Introduction

- An accurate diagnosis of PAH can be made only by RHC and so the true prevalence of PAH is unknown but is estimated at between 15–50 subjects per million in the Western world. The prevalence of PAH in different subgroups is also unclear. The lack of epidemiological data can be explained by the general lack of awareness among clinicians of PH and PAH, and a clinical focus on the condition under management, rather than its complications. When patients are admitted to hospital with an exacerbation of heart failure, or lung diseases, (the 2 groups which account for the vast majority of cases of PH), clinicians manage and treat the main cause of the patient's symptoms, usually in accordance with guidelines, rather than investigating the consequences of the condition on the pulmonary circulation and right heart.

- In an echocardiography survey of 4579 patients 10.5% had PH. Of these 483 patients with PH, 79% had left heart disease (group 2), 10% had lung diseases and hypoxia (group 3), 4.2% had PAH (group 1), 0.6% had CTEPH (group 4), and in 7% it was not possible to define a diagnosis. Echocardiography would probably overestimate the true prevalence of PAH because it would not distinguish PAH from PH; most patients with high TVRs would not have PAH but other causes of PH.

- PAH may develop at any age from childhood to people aged over 80. 25% of cases occur after the age of 60.

- The biggest subtype of PAH is IPAH accounting for 40% of all PAH patients. The next biggest group is CTD-PAH (15%), and then congenital heart diseases (CHDs; 11%), POPH (10%), appetite suppressants (a decreasing proportion at 9%), HIV 6%, familial 4%, and others may have >1 risk factor.

- 10% of systemic sclerosis (SSc) patients develop PAH justifying the use of screening programmes using echocardiography and lung function testing annually. The prevalence of PAH in SSc and other connective tissue diseases (CTDs) may be higher than currently suspected because of lack of awareness and under-investigation of patients with vague symptoms of tiredness and mild breathlessness.

- The female : male ratio in PAH is 1.9:1 and this female predominance applies to most PAH subgroups apart from HIV and POPH. The strong female predominance in CTD, results in an even greater female : male ratio, e.g. 4:1 in systemic sclerosis.

- A small but unknown proportion of patients with PH have a contributory pulmonary vasculopathy.

- Registries also reveal that most patients (>65%) are WHO class 3 or 4 at the time of diagnosis, with an average age of 50 years; 65% of patients are 5.

Congenital heart disease-associated PAH

The commonest types of CHDs associated with PAH are atrial and ventricular septal defects and patent ductus arteriosus. Although complex CHD and Eisenmenger's syndrome are less common, PAH is more likely in these patients due to high flow and high right ventricular pressure (RVP).

Group 2: PH due to left heart disease

The majority of patients with either systolic, diastolic, or combined systolic and diastolic heart failure present with symptoms similar to those of PH patients. In all cases of chronic heart failure, including aortic and mitral valve disease, the extent of PH depends on the severity of the underlying heart problem.

Group 3: Lung diseases with or without hypoxaemia

Echocardiographic studies suggest that at least 20% of patients with at least one previous hospital admission for COPD and respiratory failure have PH. At least 50% of patients with severe COPD (sufficient to consider transplantation) have PH which is usually not severe. 40% of patients with interstitial lung disease have PH.

Group 4: CTEPH

- The prevalence and incidence of CTEPH are not clear. The incidence of PE is around 1 per 1000 of the population per year. The incidence of CTEPH following acute venous thromboembolism is estimated to be between 8–51 cases per 1 million of the population. 30% of CTEPH patients do not give a history of venous thrombosis or embolism and so 'silent' emboli in the past may trigger CTEPH in some patients.
- The incidence of CTEPH after acute pulmonary embolism has been reported at 1–4% over the first 2 years post event.
- CTEPH may be found in patients without previous acute pulmonary emboli (PE) or deep vein thrombosis (DVT).

Group 5: PH with unclear and/or multifactorial mechanisms

There are no satisfactory epidemiological data for this group.

Prevalence of PAH in subgroups

- PAH: 15–50/million
- IPAH: 6/million
- SSc: 7–12%
- HIV: 0.5%
- POPH: 2–6%
- CHD: 5–10%
- Schistosomiasis: 0.025%
- Haemolytic anaemia: <8%
- CTEPH after PEs: 4% of patients.

Epidemiology and management of PAH in PVOD and/or PCH

Epidemiology and management of PAH in PVOD and/or PCH 70

Epidemiology and management of PAH in PVOD and/or PCH

Both PVOD and PCH are rare causes of PAH. PVOD is more common than PCH. They are grouped together because their histology and clinical presentations are similar. They are thought to be part of a spectrum of IPAH and familial PAH. Their presentation and risk factors are also similar. Risk factors include scleroderma, HIV infection, and the use of anorexigens. Both PVOD and PCH may be familial. As in IPAH and familial PAH, *BMPR2* mutations occur in PVOD.

Several features of PVOD and PCH, however, are different from IPAH and familial PAH. These include:
- Lung crackles and finger clubbing.
- Computed tomography (CT) chest findings of ground glass opacities, septal thickening, and mediastinal adenopathy.
- Lower CO transfer factor.
- Lower oxygen saturation.

Generally, the responses of PVOD and PCH to PAH therapies are not as good as other forms of PAH; some patients develop pulmonary oedema on these therapies.

Isolated case reports suggest benefit using sildenafil, while case series have suggested transient benefit with bosentan in individuals with histologically proven PVOD. Thus in these conditions there is little evidence for monotherapy let alone combination therapy. Current advice is to consider patients with disproportionate symptoms, findings of right heart failure despite modestly elevated pressures, or those with a poor response to therapy for lung biopsy.

PVOD and PCH are rarities, of importance because of the resistance to current therapeutic agents. Mishandled, these conditions can lead to acute pulmonary oedema during vasodilator testing and during treatment with prostanoids.

Drugs and toxins and PAH

Introduction 72
Definite risk factors for PAH 72
Likely risk factors for PAH 72
Possible risk factors for PAH 72
Unlikely risk factors for PAH 72

Introduction

A risk factor is defined as any substance, or condition suspected to predispose to or facilitate the development of PAH. Risk factors are graded as definite, likely, possible, or unlikely based on their association with PAH and their causal role.

Definite risk factors for PAH

- A 'definite' association is defined as an epidemic which occurred with appetite suppressants in the 1960s. The diet tablets were:
  - Fenfluramine
  - Phenylpropanolamine
  - Benfluorex
  - Aminorex
  - Dexfenfluramine.
- Use of aminorex resulted in the 1960s epidemic of PAH. Together with toxic rapeseed oil, these drugs are classified as definite risk factors. Fenfluramine-associated PAH shares clinical, functional, haemodynamic, and genetic features with IPAH. This suggests that fenfluramine is a trigger for PAH.

Likely risk factors for PAH

A single-centre, case–control study would constitute evidence for a likely risk factor. Examples are amphetamines, L-tryptophan, and methamphetamines (a very likely risk factor).

Possible risk factors for PAH

- A 'possible' association is defined as drugs with similar mechanisms of action as those in the 'definite' or 'likely' categories but which have not yet been studied (e.g. drugs to treat attention deficit disorder [ADD]).
- Possible causes of PAH include cocaine, phenylpropanolamine (found in some over-the-counter antiobesity formulations), St John's Wort, chemotherapeutic agents, and selective serotonin reuptake inhibitors when given during pregnancy.

Unlikely risk factors for PAH

- 'Unlikely' is defined as a drug which has been studied in epidemiological studies and an association with PAH has not been shown:
  - Oral contraceptives, oestrogen, cigarette smoking.

PAH associated conditions

19	CTD-associated PAH	**75**
20	PAH associated with HIV	**87**
21	PAH associated with portal hypertension (portopulmonary hypertension)	**93**
22	PAH associated with congenital systemic-to-pulmonary cardiac shunts	**99**
23	PAH associated with schistosomiasis	**105**
24	PAH associated with chronic haemolytic anaemias	**109**

CTD-associated PAH

Introduction 76
Systemic sclerosis (scleroderma) 79
Systemic lupus erythematosus 81
Sjögren's syndrome 86
Polymyositis and dermatomyositis 86

Introduction

- SSc-PAH is the most common type of CTD-PAH (76% of all CTD-PAH cases).
- PAH is more common in limited-SSc (LSSc) vs diffuse-SSc (DSSc).
- SSc-PAH is the 2nd most common type of PAH after IPAH (15% of all PAH cases).
- PAH is much less common in systemic lupus erythematosus (SLE), dermatomyositis and polymyositis, primary Sjögren's syndrome, rheumatoid arthritis. It is more common in mixed CTD (MCTD) which combines features of SLE, SSc, and/or polymyositis. Anti-RNP (ribonuclear protein) antibody is typically present in MCTD.

Pathology of CTD-PAH

The histology of CTD-PAH is virtually identical to IPAH but the pulmonary veins are more frequently involved.

The pathophysiological mechanisms resulting in CTD-PAH are unclear. The presence of ANA, rheumatoid factor (RhF), immunoglobulin G (IgG), and complement deposits in the pulmonary vessels suggest an immune-mediated mechanism.

Prevalence of PAH in CTD

The prevalence of PAH in CTD has been estimated from echocardiography and depends on the tricuspid velocity (TV) value used and whether patients have associated pulmonary fibrosis. In the absence of severe pulmonary fibrosis, the prevalence of PAH in catheter-based studies in SSc is 8%.

CTD-PAH and screening

- Annual screening for PAH in SSc patients is performed with clinical assessment, echocardiography, and pulmonary function tests (PFTs). The yield in symptom-free patients is lower than in symptomatic patients.
- Epidemiological data relying solely on echocardiographic estimates of PAP are inaccurate.
- The cut-off TVR value used determines the sensitivity and specificity of echocardiography in screening. There is a false positive rate of 45% using a TVR of >3.0m/s in symptom-free SSc patients or a TVR of 2.5–3.0m/s in breathless patients.
- Patients discovered to have PAH should be screened for CTD which should be characterized.

Clinical features of CTD-PAH

In the early stages, PAH patients are usually symptom free. Early symptoms are non-specific and include breathlessness and fatigue which may lead patients to ignore them or reduce their activities because they feel that they are simply unfit or suffering from a viral infection. GPs may attribute the symptoms to stress or overwork, or to a cardiorespiratory disease or asthma. Referral to a chest physician or cardiologist should prompt a request for echocardiography which should alert the specialist to the diagnosis of PAH.

Immunology and antibody profiles in CTD-PAH

Rheumatoid factor +ve in (%)
- Sjögren's syndrome: ≤100
- RA: 70–80
- SLE: ≤40
- SSc: 30
- Normal controls: 5–10.

Antinuclear antibodies (ANA)+ve in (%)
- SLE: 95
- Sjögren's syndrome: 68
- SSc: 64
- RA: 32
- Normal controls: 0–2.

RHC and diagnosis of PAH in SSc

RHC is essential for diagnosis. There are some caveats:
- The PCWP may be high in SSc patients with lung diseases with big respiratory 'swings', giving a misleading diagnosis of post-capillary PH.
- The PCWP may be falsely low in dehydrated patients despite left ventricular diastolic dysfunction (LVDD).
- The LVEDP should be measured if there is doubt about the accuracy of the PCWP.
- PVR is no longer a criterion for diagnosing PAH as this can be misleading. The PVR will be identical in patients with the same cardiac output if one has a mPAP of 28mmHg and PCWP of 14mmHg (TPG 14mmHg), and the other a mPAP of 18mmHg and PCWP of 4mmHg (TPG 14mmHg). Repeat RHC may be required to identify those patients with progressive changes in the pulmonary microcirculation.
- The majority of SSc are 'middle aged'. Coronary artery disease (CAD) should not be overlooked as a cause of LVDD and a raised PCWP. Myocardial ischaemia may be precipitated by pulmonary vasodilators.
- The mPAP may be spuriously low in severe SSc-PAH due to RV failure and a failure to generate an appropriate RV systolic pressure. A high RA and RVEDP ≥10mmHg indicate RV dysfunction.

Vasodilator testing in SSc-PAH

The role of acute vasodilator studies remains unclear in SSc-PAH. <10% of CTD patients may have an acute vasodilator response, but a long-term response to calcium channel blockers (CCBs) is exceptionally rare. Vasodilator testing is almost certainly not worthwhile in SSc-PAH.

Prognosis in CTD-PAH

The prognosis of CTD-PAH is worse than IPAH. The unadjusted comparative risk of death in CTD-PAH vs IPAH is 2.9. The reduced survival of CTD-PAH patients is due to the predominance of SSc-PAH which is associated with co-morbidities including modest lung fibrosis, GI involvement, renal impairment, and myocardial fibrosis.
- The prognosis of SSc-PAH has improved over recent years with current therapies but remains poor. Survival at 1 and 3 years is 78% and 47% respectively. PAH is the major cause of premature death in SSc.

- Survival is even worse (28% at 3 years) if SSc-PAH is associated with lung fibrosis.
- Acute SSc renal impairment is unusual but an adverse prognostic finding.
- Prognosis in PAH is determined by RV function and the ability of the RV to respond to ↑ workload. The prognosis of SSc-PAH is generally worse than other forms of PAH due to associated heart and lung disease and other comorbidities.
- In scleroderma with myocardial involvement, the RV response to increasing PAPs is blunted. RV failure and a fall in CO occur at lower PAP. Magnetic resonance imaging (MRI) of the heart in SSc-PAH may show areas of myocardial fibrosis.
- Survival of PAH associated with CTDs other than SSc is similar to IPAH.

Mechanisms of PH in SSc

A high mPAP in SSc may be due to:
- PAH with proliferative pulmonary vasculopathy.
- Lung fibrosis due to prominent parenchymal destruction. Patients with SSc and severe lung fibrosis are not known to benefit from targeted therapy.
- Post-capillary pulmonary hypertension due to LV diastolic and systolic dysfunction resulting from myocardial fibrosis.
- PVOD due to the more diffuse nature of the vascular lesions associated with scleroderma.
- Or any combination of these.

Identifying the causes of PH in CTD

- It is difficult to quantitate the individual contributions to the high PAP because there is no clear haemodynamic relationship between the extent of lung fibrosis or LVDD, and mPAP. Quantifying the extent of lung fibrosis from respiratory function tests (RFTs) or high-resolution CT (HRCT) lung scans is difficult.
- Each of these various factors may be present to different degrees in SSc or may become dominant over time. It is important to characterize the main drivers of PH in each patient. The results from RHC, echocardiography, MRI, lung function testing, and HRCT lung scanning provide complementary information to confirm and characterize the pathophysiology.
- CTED-PH must also be excluded with V/Q scanning or CTPA or invasive pulmonary angiography.

Further reading

Baker DM, Denton C. Vascular complications of systemic sclerosis: A molecular perspective. In: D Abraham, C Handler, M Dashwood, *et al.* (eds). *Vascular Complications in Human Disease: Mechanisms and Consequences*, pp. 119–27. London: Springer; 2008.

Coghlan JG, Handler C. Connective tissue disease associated pulmonary arterial hypertension. *Lupus* 2006; **15**:138–42.

Mukerjee D, St George D, Coleiro B, et al. Prevalence and outcome in systemic sclerosis associated pulmonary arterial hypertension: application of a registry approach. *Ann Rheum Dis* 2003; **62**:1088–93.

Systemic sclerosis (scleroderma)

Systemic sclerosis (SSc), or scleroderma, is a multisystem, immunologically-mediated condition. It is characterized by skin fibrosis, prominent vascular involvement causing Raynaud's syndrome, gut involvement with reflux, dysphagia, and bowel disturbance, life-threatening renal crises with acute renal failure, subclinical myocardial fibrosis and ischaemia, lung fibrosis, and PH.

There are two main forms of SSc:
- *Limited SSc* (LSSc, skin involvement distal to elbows and knees plus the face), formerly called CREST syndrome which highlights some of the conditions comprising limited SSc:
  - Calcinosis of the subcutaneous tissues
  - Raynaud's
  - oEsophageal and gut dysmotility
  - Sclerodactyly
  - Telangiectasia.
  - >60% of scleroderma patients have the limited form.
- *Diffuse SSc* (DSSc, skin thickening extends proximally to the elbows and knees)

Lung fibrosis and renal crises are more frequent in diffuse SSc compared to limited SSc. Scl-70 antibodies are associated with lung involvement, cardiac and renal changes. The prognosis of diffuse SSc is usually worse than limited SSc.

Clinical features of SSc
- *Skin thickening:* characteristically in the fingers (sclerodactyly), but may extend proximally (beyond the elbows or knees) and affect the entire body (DSSc). Leads to contractures of the fingers with loss of dexterity.
- *Raynaud's:* triphasic colour changes of the fingers and toes. In SSc this may be associated with digital ulcers. Vascular changes are evident in the nail-fold capillaries. Associated medial thickening in the small digital vessels may lead to severe ischaemia with gangrene, or ischaemic resorption of the distal phalanx, and autoamputation. Raynaud's often precedes SSc by several years.
- *Telangiectasia:* more common in LSSc, often present on the face, fingers.
- *Calcinosis:* subcutaneous calcium deposits are common and may progress to troublesome digital ulceration, especially when ischaemia or infection is present.
- *Oesophageal dysmotility:* dysphagia and acid reflux are common and troublesome. It is treated with H2-blockers and other drugs. Reflux and aspiration may aggravate pulmonary fibrosis and commonly contraindicates lung transplantation. All scleroderma patients are assessed with oesophageal studies to assess reflux before being accepted for heart/lung transplantation to treat PAH.
- *Pulmonary involvement:* most commonly pulmonary fibrosis.
- *Gastrointestinal involvement:* stasis-associated bacterial overgrowth and incontinence, constipation and/or diarrhoea and bloating.

- *Renal involvement*: renal crises, present as acute renal failure often associated with severe hypertension. Renal crises occur mainly in patients with DSSc and during the first few years of the disease. Steroid therapy is a recognized risk factor for renal crises.
- *Cardiac and pericardial involvement*: clinically significant pericardial effusions and myocarditis occur rarely. Diastolic dysfunction is comparatively common, probably related to mid-LV wall fibrosis.

Immunological testing in SSc

- Anticentromere, dsDNA, anti-Rho, U3-RNP, B23, Th/To, and U1-RNP antibodies may be positive in LSSc.
- U3-RNP antibodies are associated with DSSc. The pathogenetic role of antibodies in SSc-PAH is not defined.

LFTs

LFTs are used to assess the presence of:
- Significant COPD which should be treated.
- Lung fibrosis (proportionate reduction in TLC and FVC).
- Disproportionate reduction in DLCO with normal TLC, suggesting PAH.

Caution: the normal range of FVC is 70–130% of predicted. Therefore, significant lung disease may be present with 'normal' lung function. Lung function may be abnormal despite well-preserved parenchymal architecture on HRCT scanning. Although rare, PVOD is a cause of PAH and should be excluded with an HRCT lung scan but is typically associated with severe reductions in gas transfer.

Management issues in SSc-PAH

Our current policy is to treat aggressively all evidence of internal organ involvement, often with cyclophosphamide, followed by steroid and aza-thioprine maintenance. Pulmonary pressures rarely fall in response to immunosuppression.

These differences aside, treatment is as for IPAH. Importantly, response to immunosuppression is sufficiently uncertain that standard treatment (ERA, PDE-5 inhibition, and prostanoids) should not be delayed.

Another important consideration is that these are multisystem diseases, thus very few of these patients will be accepted for transplantation. This alters the approach to end-stage patients, where the focus is on palliation rather than work-up for transplantation.

Further reading

Clements PJ. Systemic sclerosis (scleroderma) and related disorders: clinical aspects. *Baillieres Best Pract Res Clin Rheumatol* 2000; **12**:1–16.

Systemic lupus erythematosus

Pathobiology of SLE

SLE is a non-organ-specific autoimmune disease. Antibodies are produced against a variety of autoantigens (e.g. ANA) in 95% of patients. High titre of antibodies against double-stranded DNA (ds-DNA) is almost virtually diagnostic of SLE.

Immunopathology results in polyclonal B-cell secretion of pathogenic autoantibodies and subsequent formation of immune complexes which deposit in various sites, notably the kidneys.

Prevalence and epidemiology of SLE

SLE is 9× more common in ♀ compared to ♂. The prevalence is 0.2% and it is more common in Afro-Caribbeans, Asians, and in those who are HLA B8, DR2, or DR3 +ve. 10% of relatives of patients with SLE are affected.

Diagnosis of SLE

SLE is a relapsing and remitting illness with peak age at onset at 30–40 years. Constitutional symptoms including fatigue, malaise, oral ulcers, arthralgia, photosensitive skin rashes, lymphadenopathy, pleuritic chest pains, headache, paraesthesiae, symptoms of dry eyes and mouth, Raynaud's phenomenon, and mild hair loss are more likely presentations than the well-described young woman with joint pains and a malar rash. There is often considerable delay before the diagnosis is considered in patients with low-grade disease. Prognosis is dependent on early diagnosis which is based on a full clinical assessment.

Renal involvement (lupus nephritis) presents insidiously, and if it is not detected early, the risk of progression to renal impairment is high.

SLE can be safely diagnosed if 4 or more of the following 11 criteria are present, serially or simultaneously (but note not all lupus patients will meet these standardized diagnostic criteria):

- 1. Malar rash (butterfly) on the face, fixed erythema, flat or raised over the face but sparing the nasolabial folds.
- 2. Discoid rash: erythematous raised patches with follicular plugging and atrophic scarring. The erythema on the face, ears, forehead, and chest progresses to pigmented hyperkeratotic oedematous papules and then atrophic depressed lesions.
- 3. Photosensitivity.
- 4. Oral ulcers.
- 5. Arthritis: joint involvement occurs in 90% of patients; a non-erosive arthritis involving 2 or more peripheral joints with tenderness, swelling, or effusion. Aseptic bone necrosis may occur.
- 6. Serositis:
  - Pleuritis, lung function abnormalities in 80%, pleural effusion.
  - Pericarditis with ECG changes, pericardial rub, or effusion.
- 7. Renal disease:
  - a) Persistent proteinuria (>0.5g/d, 3+ on dipstix).
  - b) Cellular casts (red cell, granular, or mixed).
- 8. CNS disorders:

- a) Seizures with no other identifiable cause.
- b) Psychosis with no other identifiable cause.
- 9. Haematological problems:
  - a) Haemolytic anaemia with reticulocytosis.
  - b) Leucopenia (WBC <4 × 10^9/L).
  - c) Lymphopenia (<1500 × 10^9).
  - d) Thrombocytopenia (<100 × 10^9/L) for no other reasons.
- 10. Immunological disorders:
  - a) Anti-DNA antibody to native DNA or
  - b) Anti-Sm antibody to Sm nuclear antigen or
  - c) Antiphospholipid antibody +ve
- 11. ANA: positive in 95% of patients.

Physical signs in SLE

Criteria as for diagnosis plus: fever, splenomegaly, lymphadenopathy, alopecia, recurrent abortion, retinal exudates, pulmonary oedema, fibrosing alveolitis, myalgia, anorexia, myositis, migraine, raised erythrocyte sedimentation rate (ESR) with often normal C-reactive protein (CRP).

Monitoring activity in SLE

An increase in constitutional symptoms and/or ESR, levels of complement c3↓, c4↓, c3d↑; ds-DNA antibody titres, BP, urinalysis, U&E, FBC.

Organ complications

Physicians managing patients with lupus must be alert for many potential complications in particular:

- Neuropsychiatric lupus: which may present insidiously or dramatically and can mimic almost any neurological condition.
- Lupus hepatitis: elevations of transaminases are common and can parallel disease activity. Many drugs are hepatotoxic, so confusion may arise.
- Haematological complications range from anaemic of chronic disease, through hypoplastic cytopenias (mirroring disease activity) to autoimmune cytopenias.
- Lupus nephritis is common and serious, monitoring of urinary protein and BP is mandatory at visits.
- Pulmonary complications include shrinking lung syndrome (diaphragmatic weakness), pulmonary fibrosis, PH, PE, pleurisy, pleural effusions and infection associated with immunosuppression (usually therapeutic).
- Cardiac manifestations include pericarditis, pericardial effusions, myocarditis, MI, and valve lesions.

Antiphospholipid syndrome (APS)

Antiphospholipid syndrome is a syndrome in its own right and may complicate various autoimmune disorders. Primary APS rarely progresses to SLE. It should be considered in ♀ with previous morbidity in pregnancy or thrombotic events. Severe and sometimes fatal APS occurs in 1% of lupus patients. When occurring in patients with SLE it considerably increases the risk of morbidity and death. It should be considered when SLE occurs with 1 or more of the following features:

- Arterial (with IgG or IgM antiphospholipid antibodies +ve), or venous thrombosis (lupus anticoagulant +ve)
- Thrombocytopenia
- Livedo reticularis
- Rash
- Stroke
- Adrenal haemorrhage
- Migraine
- Recurrent miscarriages
- Myelitis
- MI
- Multi-infarct dementia
- Cardiolipin antibodies.

Hughes syndrome is a distinct coagulopathy with heart valve disease. The condition is treated with long-term warfarin.

Treatment remains controversial in terms of the level of anticoagulation required to prevent recurrent thromboses. Clinical trials suggest that for most patients with recurrent venous thrombotic events a target international normalized ratio (INR) of 2.0–3.0 provides reasonable protection against further thrombosis with a low risk of bleeding. Patients at high risk of recurrent arterial thrombosis may continue to need higher target ratios of 3.0–4.5. Precise control is critical in this prothrombotic condition.

Treatment of SLE
- Non-steroidal anti-inflammatory drugs (NSAIDs), and sun-blockers for skin photosensitivity.
- Hydroxychloroquine is a mainstay of treatment (risk of irreversible retinopathy)
- High-dose prednisolone for severe episodes, combined with cyclophosphamide or steroid-sparing drugs including azathioprine, methotrexate, or mycophenolate.
- Low-dose steroids for chronic disease.
- Cyclophosphamide for nephritic disease.
- Renal transplantation for severe nephritis and renal failure.

Arthralgia and skin rashes
Isolated cutaneous lupus, including discoid lupus, is unlikely to progress to systemic disease and often responds to topical therapies. Weak topical steroid preparations in combination with hydroxychloroquine are often useful. More recently, topical preparations of tacrolimus and pimecrolimus have shown benefit in small open case series.

- Simple analgesics rather than non-steroidal anti-inflammatory agents should be used to reduce renal, cardiovascular and gastrointestinal side effects. COX2 selective agents are generally considered as contraindicated because of the potential cardiovascular risks.
- Hydroxychloroquine remains the mainstay for patients with mild SLE, especially for those with arthralgia, skin rashes, alopecia, and oral or genital ulceration. It is well tolerated, disease-modifying and has a weak antithrombotic action. Its beneficial effects on serum lipids and

blood glucose and its effects in reducing the risk of cataracts make it especially useful in patients who also need long-term corticosteroids.
- Mepacrine in low dose and added on to hydroxychloroquine is another safe antimalarial and is useful in mild SLE. Ocular toxicity is rare and, providing there is no major renal impairment and vision is checked annually, long-term antimalarial therapy is relatively safe. No blood monitoring is needed, but patients should be warned about the risk of skin rashes, which may occur in 5–10% of patients and resolve on withdrawal.

Lupus nephritis

Short courses of low-dose pulsed cyclophosphamide followed by azathioprine achieve similar results to a high-dose regime with less toxicity. Mycophenolate mofetil may be useful as both induction and maintenance therapy for severe proliferative lupus nephritis and may eventually supersede the use of cyclophosphamide for most patients.

Central nervous system disease

Central nervous system (CNS) disease in lupus has several manifestations from seizures to psychosis. Neuropsychiatric manifestations attributable to APS include strokes, seizures, movement disorders, transverse myelopathy, demyelination syndromes, transient ischaemic attacks, cognitive dysfunction, visual loss, and headaches including migraine.

Prognosis of SLE

Patients, particularly those diagnosed early and without major complications, may have a normal lifespan. It is difficult to predict which patients will progress to severe multisystem disease with a poor outcome. Morbidity and mortality are generally higher in patients with extensive multisystem disease and multiple autoantibodies. Prognosis ultimately depends on the amount of damage (permanent scars or irreversible organ dysfunction) accrued over the course of the disease. Treatment therefore aims to eliminate inflammation and thrombosis, minimizing damage. Accelerated atherosclerosis is now recognized as a major contributor to premature death through MI and cerebrovascular disease.

SLE and PH

- Compared to SSc-PAH, SLE-PAH appears to be much less frequent (around 1%). It may be associated with antiphospholipid antibodies.
- Lupus patients are generally younger than scleroderma patients.
- SLE has multiple potential mechanisms for producing PH, including:
  - Pulmonary vasculitis and chronic low grade inflammation
  - Recurrent thromboembolic disease and pulmonary embolism due to antiphospholipid syndrome
  - Lung fibrosis and shrinking lung fibrosis. Direct or indirect cardiac involvement causing post-capillary PH appears to be rare.

SLE and CTEPH

Significant PH due to inappropriate organization of PE can be treated with thromboendarterectomy and long-term warfarin.

Management of SLE-PAH

- The activity of the SLE determines the severity and course of associated PAH. PAH deteriorates with SLE flare-ups and subsides when the SLE remits and so control of lupus activity is paramount. Lupus patients often suffer from general debility. With acute flare-ups there may be: photophobia, joint pain and restriction of movement, rashes, serositis, neurological and renal involvement and buccal ulceration, which need identification and management.
- Acute lupus flare-ups lead to worsening of PAH. Aggressive immunosuppression is important and often sufficient to control deterioration in PAH, without the need for additional PAH-targeted therapies. A good response to high-dose immunosuppressive therapy usually results in improvement in SLE-PAH.
- The indications for treatment of SLE-PAH are the same as for other types of PAH.

Further reading

D'Cruz DP. Systemic lupus erythematosus. *BMJ* 2006; **332**:890–4.

Sjögren's syndrome

- PAH is only very occasionally seen in primary Sjögren's syndrome.
- Typical symptoms include sicca syndrome of dry eyes, and dry mouth. There may also be dyspareunia, dry skin, dysphagia, otitis media, and pneumonia.
- It may also be associated with peripheral neuropathy, thrombocytopenia, leucopenia, and vasculitis. Lymphocyte and plasma cell infiltration of the salivary glands is the rule; this may also be seen in the lungs and liver.
- There is a strong association with other CTDs (rheumatoid in up to 50%).
- Diagnosis: Schirmer's test showing reduced tear production. Anti-Ro and anti-La antibodies are commonly present.
- Treatment: artificial tears, drinks.
- Anti-TNF (tumour necrosis factor) and topical interferon are being trialled for systemic disease.

Polymyositis and dermatomyositis

Clinical features

- Symmetrical proximal muscle weakness and inflammation. Muscle involvement may result in: dysphagia, dysphonia, facial oedema, and respiratory weakness may occur.
- 9–23% of cases are associated with internal malignancy.

Signs

Macular rash (dermatomyositis) over back and shoulders, lilac/purple rash on face, red papules on extensor surfaces of fingers (Gottron's papules), rough cracked skin of hands (mechanic's hands), fever, Raynaud's, lung involvement, polyarthritis/arthralgia, calcifications, retinitis, myocarditis, dysphagia, and gut dysmotility.

Diagnosis

- Raised ALT and creatine kinase, electromyography (EMG), and muscle biopsy.
- Anti-Jo1 antibodies may be present and associated with alveolitis and lung fibrosis.

Chapter 20

PAH associated
with HIV

Epidemiology of HIV 88
Virology and immunology 88
Stages of HIV infection 88
Management of HIV 89
HIV and PH 89
Diagnosis of HIV-PAH 90
Prognosis 90
Treatment of HIV-PAH 90
Further reading 91

Epidemiology of HIV

The majority of people with HIV are in Africa. The prevalence worldwide is thought to be >40 million. The UK incidence is >4400/year. Sexual contact accounts for 75% of cases (heterosexual as frequent as homosexual infection), the rest by infected blood products, IV drug abuse, and perinatal infection.

AIDS (acquired immunodeficiency syndrome) is defined as the presence of one or more AIDS defining illnesses plus evidence of HIV infection and is one end of a spectrum of disease caused by HIV.

Virology and immunology

HIV-1 and HIV-2 are RNA retroviruses causing AIDS. HIV binds to CD4 receptors on helper T lymphocytes, monocytes, macrophages, and neural cells. The CD4+ve cells migrate to lymphoid tissue and the virus replicates to form billions of new virions, which infect new CD4+ cells. The CD4+ cells become functionally incompetent leading to immune dysfunction. The number of circulating viruses (viral load) predicts progression to AIDS.

Stages of HIV infection

- 1. Acute infection: may be no symptoms.
- 2. Seroconversion: transient illness (flu-like illness, with rash, and rarely meningoencephalitis) 2–6 weeks after HIV infection. Clinical picture similar to infectious mononucleosis.
- 3. Asymptomatic infection with some patients having generalized lymphadenopathy (PGL), lasting for >3 months.
- 4. Followed by the non-specific symptoms of AIDS-related complex (ARC) of fever, night sweats, diarrhoea, weight loss. Opportunistic infection with oral *Candida*, herpes zoster, herpes simplex, seborrhoeic dermatitis, fungal infections. This is a prodrome to AIDS.
- 5. AIDS is HIV infection with a CD4 count $<200 \times 10^6$/L and 'indicator diseases' including:
  - *Pulmonary infections:* various including *Pneumocystis jiroveci* (previously called *P. carinii*), atypical presentations of pyogenic pneumonias, *Mycobacterium tuberculosis*, fungi, cytomegalovirus, Kaposi's sarcoma, lymphoma, *M. avium* intracellulare (MAI).
  - *Cardiovascular:* dilated cardiomyopathy, pericarditis, non-infectious thrombotic endocarditis, accelerated atherosclerosis, PAH.
  - *Gut:* oral and oesophageal *Candida*, herpes simplex, aphthous ulcers, tumours. Anorexia and weight loss. Abnormal LFTs and hepatomegaly. Sclerosing cholangitis, MAI syndrome including fever, night sweats, malaise, anorexia, weight loss, abdominal pain, diarrhoea, hepatomegaly, anaemia, perianal disease.

- *Neurological:* acute HIV meningoencephalitis, myelopathy, peripheral neuropathy. Chronic HIV causing dementia, meningitis, CMV encephalitis, cryptococcal meningitis.
- *Tumours:* cerebral lymphoma, B-cell non-Hodgkin's lymphoma.
- *Eye:* CMV retinitis in 45% of AIDS cases causing ↓ acuity and, sometimes, blindness.
- *Tuberculosis:* a very serious complication.
- *Leishmaniasis.*
- *Kaposi's sarcoma.*

Management of HIV

- Referral to a specialized HIV unit is recommended.
- Life expectancy in HIV has improved due to highly effective antiretroviral therapy and aggressive early treatment of opportunistic infections.

HIV and PH

- The prevalence in patients is reported at around 0.5% and the incidence is thought to be falling with triple therapy of the infection. The proportion of a given population of PAH patients due to HIV depends on the prevalence of HIV and the aggression with which these patients are screened.
- HIV represents 7% of cases of PAH. PAH occurs in around 1 in 200 cases of HIV infection and is more common in men.
- The histology, clinical presentation, haemodynamic findings, and histological appearances of HIV-associated PAH are similar to IPAH. The mechanism is unclear.
- HIV virus has not been found in pulmonary vessels and so the virus may cause PAH indirectly through secondary messengers, e.g. cytokines, growth factors, endothelin, or viral proteins.
- Inflammation plays a part in HIV-PAH with signs of chronic inflammation, immune activation and dysregulation with release of cytokines and growth factors. There is ↑ expression of PDGF, a potent stimulus for SMC and fibroblast growth and migration, and VEGF produced by T cells increasing vascular permeability and endothelial cell proliferation.

Diagnosis of HIV-PAH

- The clinical presentation is similar to IPAH. The majority of patients are in WHO (World Health Organization) classes III or IV at the time of diagnosis.
- HIV may be diagnosed as part of the diagnostic work-up for patients with chronic hepatitis B or C, exposure to drugs and toxins, or pulmonary emboli in IV drug abusers. Most patients with HIV-PAH are ♂ drug abusers.
- Screening for PAH in symptom-free HIV-infected patients is not recommended.
- Echocardiography should be done in symptomatic patients with unexplained dyspnoea to detect possible cardiovascular complications.
- RHC should be done if the TVR is raised above 2.8m/s. Vasoreactivity testing is not recommended and so this group of patients are not treated with CCBs.

Prognosis

- When first described, HIV-PAH had a prognosis similar to PVOD, however, due to the excellent response to pulmonary vasodilator therapy and improved antiviral therapy, prognosis in this group is generally better than in IPAH.
- Prognosis depends on mPAP and RV function.
- Treatment: most patients are well controlled on effective stabilization of HIV with antiretroviral treatment plus simple oral pulmonary vasodilator therapy.

Treatment of HIV-PAH

There have been only small numbers of HIV patients included in PAH trials and these have been open-label. There is little evidence from randomized controlled trials (RCTs) to support best management in HIV-PAH.

Optimal management of the HIV is pivotal but insufficient once PAH has developed.

ERAs

Bosentan improved functional capacity and haemodynamics in the only RCT performed. Long-term registry data shows that prognosis is very substantially improved compared with historical controls in patients treated with bosentan. Hepatic tolerability of ERAs is similar to other forms of PAH. As in other cases, bosentan is contraindicated if there is advanced liver disease (Child–Pugh class C).

Sildenafil

Sildenafil is metabolized by cytochrome P(CYP)450 3A4 and interacts with antiretrovirals, particularly protease inhibitors, increasing the sildenafil blood level, and so the dose of sildenafil should be reduced. It is contraindicated with potent CYP3A4 inhibitors including ritonavir.

Sildenafil has been shown equally effective in reducing PVR in HIV associated PAH as prostanoids, whether this will lead to similar improvements in survival as seen with bosentan is as yet unclear.

Prostanoids

IV prostanoids significantly improve exercise capacity and haemodynamics but there is a risk of infection and thromboembolism, particularly in this immunosuppressed group. There is also concern about using an IV line in patients who may continue to abuse drugs. Nebulized prostanoids avoid these practical concerns but there is little evidence so far to support their use.

Warfarin

Warfarin is not usually recommended because HIV patients have an ↑ bleeding risk, and there may be problems with compliance and other drug interactions.

Further reading

Cohen MS, Shaw GM, McMichael AJ, *et al.* Acute HIV-1 infection. *N Engl J Med* 2011; **364**:1943–54.

Hammer SM. Clinical practice. Management of newly diagnosed HIV infection. *N Engl J Med* 2005; **353**:1702–10.

Opravil M, Pechère M, Speich R, *et al.* HIV associated primary pulmonary hypertension. A case control study. Swiss HIV Cohort Study. *Am J Respir Crit Care Med* 1997; **155**:990–5.

PAH associated with portal hypertension (portopulmonary hypertension)

Introduction 94
Classification of portal hypertension 94
Pathophysiology of POPH 94
Screening for POPH 95
Clinical presentation 95
Haemodynamics in POPH 95
Diagnosis of POPH 95
Medical treatment of POPH 96
Prognosis of POPH 97
Further reading 97

Introduction

- POPH is PAH in the setting of portal hypertension.
- POPH is a portal pressure gradient (the difference in pressure between the portal vein and the hepatic veins) of 5mmHg or greater. It has become more important with the ↑ frequency of liver transplantation and its complications in patients with undiagnosed PAH.
- POPH represents between 5–16% of cases of PAH in registries. 3–9% of all liver transplant candidates have POPH.
- POPH is more common in ♀, autoimmune liver disease, and after a portocaval shunt. POPH is pathologically indistinguishable from IPAH and is characterized by the development of vasoconstriction, vascular remodelling, and thrombosis within the pulmonary vasculature.
- It is an important diagnosis to consider in liver transplant patients.
- The primary goals of therapy are to provide symptomatic relief, prolong survival, and improve pulmonary haemodynamics to facilitate safe and successful liver transplantation.

Classification of portal hypertension

- *Pre-hepatic:* portal vein thrombosis, splenic vein thrombosis.
- *Intrahepatic:* cirrhosis (80% of cases in the UK), schistosomiasis (commonest cause of portal hypertension in the world), sarcoidosis, myeloproliferative diseases, congenital hepatic fibrosis.
- *Post-hepatic:* right heart failure, Budd–Chiari syndrome, constrictive pericarditis, veno-occlusive disease.

Pathophysiology of POPH

- The mechanisms underlying POPH are unclear. Portal hypertension is thought to predispose patients to disturbances in the homeostatic regulation of numerous neurohumoral and vasoactive mediators that induce the development of PAH. Deficiencies in endothelial prostacyclin synthase, excess circulating endothelin-1, and pulmonary artery aggregates are seen in POPH. A current hypothesis is that ↑ intrahepatic liver pressure exposes the lung arteries via portosystemic collaterals to blood constituents and in genetically predisposed patients causes PAH.
- PAH occurs due to a high portal pressure rather than the underlying liver disease. POPH may occur for several reasons, including cirrhosis from any cause, or any obstruction to portal flow in the liver (e.g. portal vein thrombosis), that impedes portal flow to the liver.
- POPH is most prevalent among patients with end-stage liver disease, and its severity seems to be independent of the aetiology or severity of liver disease.

Screening for POPH

All liver transplant candidates must be screened for the presence of POPH because of the high perioperative mortality risk of liver transplantation associated with this condition. Primary screening for POPH consists of echocardiography. RHC may be necessary.

- Chest X-ray (CXR) and ECG become abnormal only in severe PAH and so are not suitable for screening due to their low sensitivity.
- All liver transplant candidates should be screened with echocardiography to estimate pulmonary artery systolic pressure (PASP) and evaluate RV function size and other parameters of RV impairment.
- RHC should be performed if PAH is suggested by echocardiography. It is estimated that around 10% of liver transplant candidates would need RHC to confirm or exclude POPH.

Clinical presentation

Signs of PAH may be masked by signs of chronic liver disease. Ascites, peripheral oedema, fatigue, and exertional breathlessness are common in portal hypertension even without PAH.

Finger clubbing and hypoxaemia suggest the hepatopulmonary syndrome of portal hypertension, pulmonary vascular dilatation, and hypoxaemia. Chest pain and syncope suggest severe PAH.

Haemodynamics in POPH

PH may occur due to:
- Cirrhosis-associated high CO.
- High PCWP due to fluid overload and renal dysfunction.
- High PCWP due to LVDD.
- Obstruction to flow in the pulmonary arterial bed.

The PVR will usually be normal in those cases due to the high CO. The PCWP may be high due to LVDD in patients with alcohol-associated heart disease.

Diagnosis of POPH

RHC is essential to characterize the condition and also to assess patients for liver transplantation.

The diagnostic criteria are:
- A clinical diagnosis of POPH.
- RHC showing:
  - mPAP >25mmHg.
  - PAOP ≤ 15mmHg
  - PVR >3 WU
  - In the setting of confirmed portal hypertension.

Medical treatment of POPH

Impaired liver function, thrombocytopenia, auto-anticoagulation, and vasodilation have contraindicated recruitment of POPH patients into ERA trials. PDE-5Is are generally preferred because liver side effects are much less likely.

- *Liver transplantation (LIVT):* LIVT offers a potential cure but is available only to those with no or only minor elevations of PVR. With a mPAP of <35mmHg and a normal CO, the mortality risk and the risk of other transplant complications is around 14%. This increases if the mPAP is >35mmHg at which level, LIVT is contraindicated. In view of this, patients are treated aggressively with PDE-5Is and with ERAs in an attempt to achieve this haemodynamic position.
- PDE-5Is may be used in an attempt to reduce the mPAP to <35mmHg, reducing the perioperative risk but there is little information on this approach.
- Beta-blockers, used to prevent variceal bleeds, may be dangerous in patients with POPH-PAH by decreasing CO, HR, and increasing PVR without lowering mPAP.
- Bosentan is generally well tolerated, however this agent is generally regarded as contraindicated if the transaminases exceed 3× normal. Ambrisentan is less frequently associated with liver function abnormalities, but there is less experience with ambrisentan.
- Anticoagulation is generally not advised in POPH because there is no evidence base (the evidence is for IPAH). Anticoagulation is unnecessary when the INR is raised due to liver disease.
  - Even where the INR is not elevated, thrombocytopenia may contribute to an adverse risk:benefit ratio for anticoagulation. If the platelet count is <80 × 10^9/L then the risks of anticoagulation increase.
- Prostanoids are used, but these have some antiplatelet effects, which can increase bleeding tendency, cause vasodilatation, which is a problem for those individuals who already have a significantly elevated CO, and when administered intravenously, increase the risk of sepsis in a population already prone to sepsis.

Prognosis of POPH

- Untreated, POPH is associated with a poor prognosis. As in other forms of PAH, death in POPH occurs due to right heart failure but also liver disease and infection.
- Without disease targeted therapies or LIVT, the 5-year survival is 14%.
- With prostanoids, the 5-year survival is 45%. The 5-year survival in non-transplanted patients has been reported as up to 68% but some patients were treated with targeted therapies. Prognosis depends on age of the patient, the presence and severity of cirrhosis, and is worse in ♀.
- LIVT has a 14% perioperative risk if the mPAP <35mmHg.
- Patients who respond to epoprostenol infusion, and other targeted therapies and who survive LIVT have a good prognosis and POPH may resolve.

Further reading

Herve P, Lebrec D, Brenot F, et al. Pulmonary vascular disorders in portal hypertension. Eur Respir J 1998; 11:1153–66.

Hoeper MM, Krowka MJ, Strassburg CP. Portopulmonary hypertension: results from a 10-year screening algorithm. Hepatology 2006; 44:1502–10.

PAH associated with congenital systemic-to-pulmonary cardiac shunts

Introduction *100*
Congenital heart disease *100*
Classification of congenital heart disease anomalies
  associated with PH *101*
Anatomical-pathophysiological classification of congenital
  systemic-to-pulmonary shunts associated with PAH *102*
Histology of CHD-PAH *104*
Medical treatment for CHD-PAH *104*
Further reading *104*

Introduction

There is an increasing number of patients with CHD-PAH due to improved surgical and medical treatments of those who have unrepaired defects. Patients should be referred to a specialist centre.

5–10% of untreated systemic-to-pulmonary shunts may lead to PAH, due to ↑ blood flow and ↑ PAP. When the right-sided pressures exceed left-sided pressures, right-to-left shunting occurs with central cyanosis (Eisenmenger syndrome).

Congenital heart disease

Risk factors identified for PAH include the size and location of the shunt. Around 6% of patients with CHD develop PAH. It is rare with ventricular septal defects (VSDs) of <1.5cm diameter (3%), but common with larger VSDs and patent ductus arteriosus (PDA, 50%). By contrast, in large atrial septal defects (ASDs) PAH occurs in <10%. Another feature of CHD-associated PAH is that the age of presentation varies with the defect—in childhood with VSDs and PDAs but in adulthood with ASDs.

Classification of congenital heart disease anomalies associated with PH

1. Lesions producing left-to-right shunts and PAH due to volume and pressure loading of the pulmonary vasculature

- Large ASD
- Large VSD
- Atrioventricular (AV) canal defect
- PDA
- Aorto-pulmonary window.

Patients with Down's syndrome are predisposed to PAH in setting of large left-to-right shunt.

Large ASDs may not cause problems until adulthood (<20% of ASD present before age 30).

Surgical aortopulmonary shunts (Potts, Blalock–Taussig, Waterson) mediate an excessive left-to-right shunt and may increase in PVR.

2. Left-sided inflow obstruction (post-capillary PH—WHO group 2)

- Obstructed pulmonary venous return
- Cor triatriatum
- Mitral stenosis
- Pulmonary vein stenosis or hypoplasia
- Aortic stenosis
- Restrictive cardiomyopathy.

3. Complex cyanotic congenital heart disease with ↑ pulmonary blood flow

- Truncus arteriosus
- Transposition of the great vessels
- Single ventricles with ↑ pulmonary blood flow.

4. Anomalies of the pulmonary arteries of veins

- Scimitar syndrome
- Tetralogy of Fallot with pulmonary atresia and major aortopulmonary collateral artery
- Total anomalous pulmonary venous return.

Anatomical-pathophysiological classification of congenital systemic-to-pulmonary shunts associated with PAH

See Table 22.1.

Table 22.1 Anatomical-pathophysiological classification of congenital systemic-to-pulmonary shunts associated with pulmonary arterial hypertension (modified from Venice 2003)

1. Type

1.1 Simple pre-tricuspid shunts

    1.1.1 Atrial septal defect (ASD)

        1.1.1.1 Ostium secundum

        1.1.1.2 Sinus venosus

        1.1.1.3 Ostium primum

    1.1.2 Total or partial unobstructed anomalous pulmonary venous return

1.2 Simple post-tricuspid shunts

    1.2.1 Ventricular septal defect (VSD)

    1.2.2 Patent ductus arteriosus

1.3 Combined shunts

    Describe combination and define predominant defect

1.4 Complex congenital heart disease

    1.4.1 Complete atrioventricular septal defect

    1.4.2 Truncus arteriosus

    1.4.3 Single ventricle physiology with unobstructed pulmonary blood flow

    1.4.4 Transposition of the great arteries with VSD (without pulmonary stenosis) and/or patent ductus arteriosus

    1.4.5 Other

2. Dimension (specify for each defect if more than one congenital heart defect exists)

2.1 Haemodynamic (specify Qp/Qs)[a]

    2.1.1 Restrictive (pressure gradient across the defect)

    2.1.2 Non-restrictive

2.2 Anatomic[b]

    2.2.1 Small to moderate (ASD ≤2.0cm and VSD ≤1.0cm)

    2.2.2 Large (ASD>2.0cm and VSD >1.0cm)

3. Direction of shunt

    3.1 Predominantly systemic-to-pulmonary

    3.2 Predominantly pulmonary-to-systemic

    3.3 Bidirectional

4. Associated cardiac and extracardiac abnormalities

5. Repair status

   5.1 Unoperated

   5.2 Palliated [specify type of operation(s), age at surgery]

   5.3 Repaired [specify type of operation(s), age at surgery]

[a]Ratio of pulmonary (Qp) to systemic (Qs) blood flow.

[b]The size applies to adult patients.

ASD, atrial septal defect; VSD, ventricular septal defect.

Reprinted from The Task Force for the Diagnosis and Treatment of Pulmonary Hypertension of the European Society of Cardiology (ESC) and the European Respiratory Society (ERS), endorsed by the International Society of Heart and Lung Transplantation (ISHLT). Guidelines for the diagnosis and treatment of pulmonary hypertension. *Eur Heart J* 2009; **30**:2493–537, with permission from Oxford University Press.

Histology of CHD-PAH

This is similar to other forms of PAH.

Medical treatment for CHD-PAH

- One trial has shown a 53m increase in the 6MWD without deterioration in arterial oxygenation and a significant reduction in PVR after a 16-week treatment period with bosentan. This was, however, a safety trial.
- Sildenafil has been used in small non-randomized studies and reduces PVR and improves functional capacity.
- Registry data suggests improved outcome in those receiving pulmonary vasodilator therapy.
- There is little information on combination therapy.
- IV prostanoids have been used and reduce PVR but the risk of thromboembolism and infection has limited their use.
- Pulmonary vasodilators do not appear to increase right-to-left shunting or cyanosis.

Further reading

Galiè N, Manes A, Palazzini M, *et al.* Management of pulmonary arterial hypertension associated with congenital systemic-to-pulmonary shunts and Eisenmenger's syndrome. *Drugs* 2008; **68**:1049–66.

Chapter 23

PAH associated with schistosomiasis

Introduction 106
Parasite life cycle 106
Diagnosis of schistosomiasis 106
Pathophysiology of schistosomiasis-associated PAH 107
Chronic schistosomiasis and PAH 107
Clinical features of schistosomiasis-PAH 107
Treatment 107

Introduction

Schistosomiasis is the 3rd leading endemic parasitic disease in the world, following malaria and amoebiasis. Schistosomiasis is believed to affect 250 million people world wide, predominantly in tropical zones of South America, Asia, and Africa. Mortality is 11,000 deaths per year.

Parasite life cycle

Schistosomiasis is caused by a group of trematode worms. The most frequent ones affecting humans are *Schistosoma mansoni* (Africa, Brazil, Venezuela, and the Caribbean), *S. haematobium* and *S. intercalatum* (Africa), *S. japonicum* (China, Indonesia, Philippines).

Among travellers to sub-Saharan Africa, who were in contact in freshwater, the rate of symptomatic infection is 55–100%.

Schistosome larvae are called cercariae which penetrate the skin of humans. They develop into schistosomula and enter capillaries and lymphatics and travel to the lungs. The worms then penetrate the alveolar-capillary membrane, ascend the bronchial tree, and travel to the gut. They migrate to the venous portal system, mature, and male and female worms unite. The worms then migrate to the mesenteric vessels and the bladder. Female worms produce eggs which pass from the lumen of blood vessels into tissues, into the bladder and bowel and are shed in the faeces or urine. The eggs hatch, releasing miricidia which infect freshwater snails. After 2 generations, the sporocysts release cercariae and the lifecycle is repeated.

1/3 of the eggs produced by *S. mansoni* and *S. japonicum* are deposited in the liver veins and cause periportal liver fibrosis and portal hypertension but not cirrhosis. Some eggs are transported to the lung capillaries.

20% of patients develop chronic schistosomiasis with hepatosplenic disease and portal hypertension.

Diagnosis of schistosomiasis

Likelihood depends on environmental exposure, and identification of eggs in the urine (*S. haematobium*) or faeces (*S. japonicum* and *S. mansoni*), or rectal biopsy (all types) and schistosomal antibodies. Liver ultrasound may show enlargement of the left lobe of the liver or periportal fibrosis.

Pathophysiology of schistosomiasis-associated PAH

Schistosome egg antigen induces an immunological reaction from the host causing a granulomatous reaction. The resulting fibro-obstructive disease occurs in the liver, intestine, and genitourinary tract but may also occur in other organs and tissues and there may multiple schistosoma granulomas in the lung parenchyma.

Whether through recurrent infiltration of the lung or by causing POPH hypertension, vascular changes in the lung arteries are similar to IPAH.

Chronic schistosomiasis and PAH

In endemic areas, e.g. Brazil, schistosomiasis accounts for 8% of cases of PAH and worldwide, possibly is the most frequent cause of PAH.

Clinical features of schistosomiasis-PAH

The presentation and management algorithm is similar to IPAH and differentiation may be difficult if there are no portal abnormalities and biopsies are negative. Serology by ELISA (enzyme-linked immunosorbent assay) is helpful in patients not from endemic areas.

Acute vasodilator testing is negative.

Treatment

Schistosomiasis-PAH

There is little evidence from RCTs that targeted therapies are helpful. CCBs are contraindicated because of portal hypertension. Anticoagulants are relatively contraindicated due to the presence of oesophageal varices and the risk of bleeding.

Schistosomiasis

Prevention has not been successful and would require major investment in the infrastructure and major societal change in endemic areas.

The effects of antiparasitic treatment are variable. Oral praziquantel effectively treats the fluke infection, but this does not reverse PH once this complication has developed.

PAH associated with chronic haemolytic anaemias

Introduction *110*
Sickle cell disease *110*
Pathophysiology of SCD *110*
Diagnosis of SCD *110*
Sickling crises (painful crisis) and the less common haemolytic, sequestration, and aplastic crises *111*
Management of sickle cell crisis *112*
Acute chest crisis *113*
Sickling and NO resistance *113*
Prevalence of PH in SCD *114*
Proposed mechanisms of PAH in SCD *114*
Pathophysiology of PH and PAH in SCD *114*
Long-term management of SCD *114*
Prevention of SCD *115*
Treatment of PAH associated with haemoglobinothies *115*

Introduction

PAH is seen most frequently in patients with sickle cell disease (SCD) compared to other haemolytic anaemias but is also associated occasionally with thalassaemia, hereditary spherocytosis, stomatocytosis, and microangiopathic haemolytic anaemia.

Sickle cell disease

- SCD (sickle cell anaemia) is a genetic, lifelong haemolytic anaemia, presenting in childhood, and common in tropical and subtropical regions where malaria is common.
- Life expectancy is reduced to an average of 42 years for ♂ and 48 years for ♀ due to renal failure, bone necrosis and osteomyelitis, iron overload due to blood transfusions, and lung complications.
- Homozygotes (HbSS) have SCD.
- Heterozygotes (HbAS) have sickle cell trait which is benign, and offers a survival advantage against falciparum malaria. Heterozygotes may also have veno-occlusive events induced by hypoxia; African patients should have a pre-op sickling test.

Pathophysiology of SCD

- 96% of normal haemoglobin (Hb) is haemoglobin A which consists of 2 alpha and 2 beta chains.
- The remainder is haemoglobin A2, which consists of 2 alpha and 2 delta chains, and haemoglobin F which consists of 2 alpha and 2 gamma chains.
- In normal HbA, glutamic acid is on the 6th position of the beta chain. In SCD, glutamic acid is replaced by valine leading to the formation of HbS and not HbA. HbA2 and HbF production are not affected.

Diagnosis of SCD

- Diagnosis is made from sampling cord blood at birth providing the opportunity for pneumococcal vaccination or penicillin V.
- Common findings: Hb= 6–8g/dL; reticulocytes 10–20% (haemolysis is variable); raised bilirubin. Blood film shows features of hyposplenism (target cells and Howell–Jolly bodies).
- Sickling of the red blood cells (RBCs), on a blood film, can be induced by the addition of sodium metabisulfite.
- Electrophoresis distinguishes SS and AS and other Hb variants. Abnormal Hb forms can be detected on Hb electrophoresis, a form of gel electrophoresis on which the various types of Hb move at varying speeds.

Sickling crises (painful crisis) and the less common haemolytic, sequestration, and aplastic crises

Triggers for sickling crises include:
- Dehydration
- Infections
- Ischaemia
- Hypoxia
- Cold
- Acidosis commonly precipitated by physical exercise.

Sometimes, no specific trigger can be identified. Most episodes of sickle cell crises last between 5–7 days.

Thrombotic or vaso-occlusive crises

These are caused by sickle-shaped RBCs that obstruct capillaries and restrict blood flow to an organ, resulting in ischaemia, pain, necrosis, and often organ damage. They may mimic pneumonia or an acute abdomen.

Many organs may be affected including:
- Brain: cerebral sickling may cause fits and focal neurological signs.
- Bone: avascular necrosis of the hip and other major joints due to thrombosis and ischaemia of bone.
- Penis: priapism and infarction of the penis.
- Kidney: acute papillary necrosis in the kidneys, chronic renal failure due to sickle cell nephropathy may result in hypertension, proteinuria, haematuria, and anaemia. If it progresses to end-stage renal failure, it carries a poor prognosis.
- Skin: leg ulcers.
- Eyes: background retinopathy, proliferative retinopathy, vitreous haemorrhages, and retinal detachments, may result in blindness. Regular annual eye checks are recommended.
- Placenta: during pregnancy, intrauterine growth retardation, spontaneous abortion.
- Lungs: acute chest syndrome results in fever, chest pain, difficulty breathing, and pulmonary infiltrates. Patients are treated for both sickling and pneumonia. Chronically, patients may develop high flow PH, post-capillary PH, lung disease-associated PH, or PAH.

The frequency, severity, and duration of these crises vary considerably.

Haemolytic crises
- These are acute accelerated drops in Hb level.
- The RBCs break down at a faster rate than the bone marrow can replace them. Haemolytic crises are particularly common in patients with coexistent G6PD deficiency.
- Management is supportive. Blood transfusions may be necessary.
- Cholelithiasis (gallstones) and cholecystitis result from excessive bilirubin production and precipitation due to prolonged haemolysis.
- Jaundice is due to the inability of the liver to remove bilirubin resulting from haemolysis.

Splenic sequestration crises

- Because of its narrow vessels and function in clearing defective RBCs, the spleen is frequently affected becoming infarcted and ineffective in childhood.
- Auto-splenectomy increases the risk of infection from encapsulated organisms. Preventive antibiotics and vaccinations are recommended.
- Splenic sequestration crises are acute, painful enlargements of the spleen due to pooling of blood.
- They need to be treated as an emergency with fluid and if necessary, blood, because patients may die within a few hours due to hypovolaemia and circulatory failure.
- The abdomen is usually bloated and very hard.

Long-term management and prophylaxis after splenic infarction

- Daily penicillin prophylaxis is used at least during childhood and often, long term. Folic acid and penicillin are given to children.
- Routine vaccination for *Haemophilus influenzae*, *Streptococcus pneumoniae*, and *Neisseria meningitidis*.

Aplastic crisis

- This is an acute deterioration in pre-existing anaemia resulting in tachycardia, fatigue, pallor, and a reduction in reticulocytes.
- This crisis may be triggered by parvovirus B19 which invades and destroys RBC precursors. In normal individuals, this is of little consequence, but the shortened RBC life of sickle-cell patients results in an abrupt, life-threatening situation.
- Reticulocyte counts drop dramatically, and the rapid turnover of RBCs leads to severe anaemia.
- Treatment is supportive; a blood transfusion may be necessary.

Management of sickle cell crisis

- Ill patients are admitted to hospital. Patients should be managed in liaison with a specialist centre.
- Give adequate, effective, usually patient-controlled analgesia, including opiates. NSAIDs (such as diclofenac or naproxen) for milder pain.
- Broad-spectrum antibiotics if there is fever.
- Rehydrate IV and keep warm.
- Give O_2 by mask for hypoxia.
- Crossmatch blood, FBC, reticulocytes, blood cultures, mid-stream specimen of urine, CXR, PCV, check liver and spleen size daily. The anaemia of the crisis is caused by haemolysis and the destruction of the red cells inside the spleen. Although the bone marrow attempts to compensate by creating new RBCs, it does not match the rate of destruction. Bone marrow transplants have been used in children.
- Blood transfusion if PCV or reticulocytes fall of if there are serious CNS or lung complications.

Acute chest crisis

- The acute chest syndrome is a serious condition with pulmonary infiltrates in complete lung segments due to fat emboli from bone marrow.
- Features include: chest pain, fever, tachypnoea, wheeze (treated with bronchodilators), and cough. Cases should be referred or discussed with a specialist unit.
- Causative organisms include *Chlamydia*, *Mycoplasma*, viruses, and also sickled RBCs.
- Ventilation may be necessary in at least 10% if PO_2 on air <9.2kPa.
- Mortality 10%.
- Red cell transfusion or exchange transfusion may be necessary.

Treatment of acute chest crisis

- Management is similar to vaso-occlusive crisis, with the addition of antibiotics e.g. a quinolone or macrolide because wall-deficient ('atypical') bacteria are thought to contribute to the syndrome.
- Oxygen is given to maintain optimal oxygenation.
- Blood transfusion or exchange transfusion (which decreases the percent of HbS in the patient's blood) may be necessary if oxygen requirements increase or the response to other measures is inadequate.
- Incentive spirometry, a technique to encourage deep breathing to minimize the development of atelectasis, is recommended.

Sickling and NO resistance

- Haemoglobin released into plasma during intravascular haemolysis scavenges NO.
- NO is continuously released by endothelium and regulates vasodilator tone, inhibits platelet and haemostatic activation, and inhibits transcriptional expression of adhesion molecules.
- The half-life of NO is short because of rapid reactions with RBC Hb to form methaemoglobin and nitrate.
- The vasodilator activity of NO is possible only because all Hb is compartmentalized in RBCs, preventing NO entering RBCs and reduces scavenging of NO with intracellular Hb.
- Hb release into plasma during haemolysis disrupts diffusion barriers and inhibits NO bioactivity leading to endothelial dysfunction and NO resistance.

Chronic NO resistance contributes to:

- Vasoconstriction.
- Proliferative vasculopathy.
- Activation of adhesion molecules, e.g. VCAM-1.
- Activation of platelets.
- Production of endothelin a vasoconstrictor and mitogen.

Prevalence of PH in SCD

- Echocardiography suggests a PAH prevalence of 20–40% in adults with SCD, but as more robust efforts are made to characterize this population with invasive evaluation the prevalence has been found to be much lower, possibly closer to 5%.
- High output states, post-capillary PH, and inaccuracy of echocardiography all contribute to the apparent differences.

Proposed mechanisms of PAH in SCD

- Haemolysis (thought to be a driver for PAH in other haemolytic anaemias) and NO scavenging.
- Oxidative stress.
- Arginine dysregulation.
- ↑ vasoactive mediators (ET-1).
- Iron overload.
- Hepatitis C.
- Liver dysfunction due to nodular regenerative hyperplasia.
- Chronic renal failure.
- Coagulopathy/thrombosis *in situ* and pulmonary emboli (CTEPH occurs in 5% of SCD patients and severe PAH).
- Splenectomy.
- Hypoxaemia with restrictive and obstructive lung disease.
- Genetic susceptibility.

Pathophysiology of PH and PAH in SCD

- The anaemia in SCD results in a high CO with a normal or modestly high PVR even in the absence of pulmonary vascular lesions.
- Cardiac impairment in HbSS can lead to pathological changes consistent with post-capillary PH.
- The histological lesions in HbSS PAH are similar to those seen in IPAH.

Long-term management of SCD

Patients should be managed in collaboration with specialist sickle cell centres.

Hydroxyurea

- Hydroxyurea was the first approved drug for the causative treatment of sickle cell anaemia.
- It reactivates fetal Hb production in place of the HbS.
- It reduces the number and severity of sickling attacks and chest syndrome, and may improve survival.
- The risks of treatment are very low.

Prevention of SCD

- Genetic counselling is important.
- Parental education prevents the majority of deaths from sequestration crises.

Treatment of PAH associated with haemoglobinothies

No adequate trials of PAH therapy have been completed in patients with haemoglobinopathy-associated PAH and so there is no evidence base for monotherapy let alone combination therapy.

Haemodynamics and treatment approaches in PH due to left heart disease

25 Haemodynamics and treatment approaches
   in PH due to left heart disease   **119**

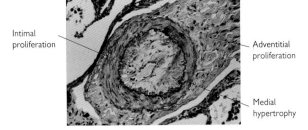

Intimal proliferation

Adventitial proliferation

Medial hypertrophy

Colour plate 1 (Also see Fig. 5.1.) A plexiform lesion in a small pulmonary arteriole showing intimal and medial disruption and hypertrophy, aneurysmal dilatation, and formation of a complex proliferative tuft of intimal cells and channels. Published with permission from S Gaine and L Rubin.

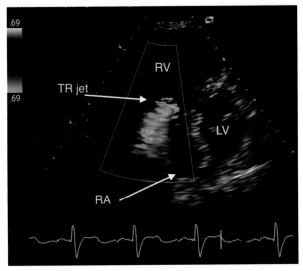

.69

.69

RV

TR jet

LV

RA

Colour plate 2 (Also see Fig. 30.10.) Short axis echocardiographic view at the level of the tricuspid valve with colour flow Doppler showing tricuspid valve regurgitation during systole. This can be used to estimate the optimal angle for determining the tricuspid gradient. LV = left ventricle. RV = right ventricle.

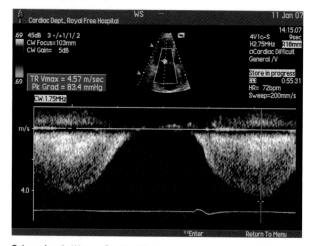

Colour plate 3 (Also see Fig. 30.11.) Estimating pulmonary pressure using echocardiography. Doppler signals are used to determine the velocity with which blood regurgitates through the tricuspid valve during systole. 70% of normal people have enough regurgitation to use this technique, the frequency is higher in PAH. Doppler relies on the change in frequency of reflected sound waves proportional to the velocity of the target. The Bernoulli equation ($P = 4V^2$ where P = pressure and V = velocity) describes this relationship. Thus the difference between right ventricular systolic pressure and right atrial systolic pressure can be directly measured. The technique is quite error prone, with a standard deviation of ±20mmHg.

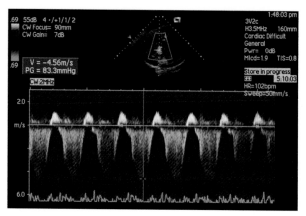

Colour plate 4 (Also see Fig. 30.19.) Tricuspid velocity assessment using Doppler. Note unless a clear envelope of regurgitant signal is available, estimates of the maximum velocity can be very inaccurate. The sweep speed should be at least 50mm/s and use of colour rather than greyscale improves the ability to see the signal. The estimate is highly angle dependent and underestimation occurs if alignment is incorrect. Overestimation may occur if the probe is causing discomfort or the patient is holding their breath in expiration causing a 'Valsalva' type phenomenon.

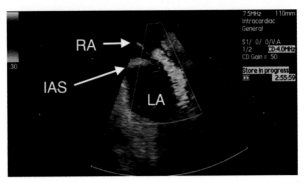

Colour plate 5 (Also see Fig. 32.1.) Intracardiac echocardiography with colour flow Doppler. A 1cm defect has been created in the intra-atrial septum (IAS), because right atrial (RA) pressure significantly exceeds left atrial (LA) pressure right-to-left flow is seen from a probe placed in the right atrium. This offloads the right ventricle while improving left ventricular filling at a cost of moderate desaturation.

Haemodynamics and treatment approaches in PH due to left heart disease

Introduction *120*
Disproportionate post-capillary PH *120*
Presentation of post-capillary PH *120*
Diagnosis of post-capillary PH *121*
Treatment of post-capillary PH *121*

Introduction

Chronic left heart failure leads to haemodynamic, autonomic, neurohumoral, and immunological abnormalities. There is activation of cytokines and inflammatory markers. It is unclear whether secondary mechanisms such as endothelial damage can result in an independent pulmonary vasculopathy in patients with heart failure.

Mechanisms responsible for the passive increase in PAP in left heart disease include:
- LVEDP increase.
- Secondary PCWP increase.
- ↑ oncotic pressure leading to hypoxia due to pulmonary oedema.

In these cases, the TPG (TPG = mPAP – PCWP) and PVR are within the normal range.

Disproportionate post-capillary PH

In a proportion of patients with heart failure the TPG is >15mmHg, the PVR is above $240d.s.cm^{-5}$, and there is a gradient between PA diastolic pressure and PCWP. Such patients are considered to have *disproportionate* PH and studies are underway to determine if treating such patients with pulmonary vasodilators is worthwhile. Caution is advised because:
- To date, most heart failure trials using pulmonary vasodilators have been negative or shown harm.
- Data from mitral stenosis surgery shows that most 'disproportionate' PH disappears with effective relief of the post-capillary load.
- Data from artificial heart devices also show resolution of disproportionate PH.
- Diuresed patients may have a relatively low PCWP at catheterization, but this may rise with effort, and pulmonary vasodilator therapy may simply promote pulmonary oedema.

Presentation of post-capillary PH

Exertional breathlessness and fatigue are the most common symptoms in all types of PH, whether pre-capillary or post-capillary. Post-capillary PH may result from LV impairment (systolic or diastolic, or both). Therefore signs of RV failure and PH (as in PAH) may be present but there will also be symptoms/signs of the underlying left heart problem.
- Angina may result from coronary heart disease causing LV impairment ('ischaemic cardiomyopathy'), a common cause of PH.
- With any cause of PH, swelling of the legs, abdominal distension, nausea, and anorexia may occur if there is RV impairment.
- Patients may have a history of hypertension, previous cardiac surgery, or known cardiac abnormality
- Risk factors may be present: diabetes, hypercholesterolaemia, smoking, FH of CAD, cardiomyopathies, premature sudden death.

- Signs of left heart disease may be present: displaced apex beat, systolic or diastolic left heart murmurs, reduced pulse volume, crackles in the lung fields.
- Rare conditions should not be forgotten: amyloid (chronic inflammatory conditions); constriction (tuberculosis, prior cardiac surgery).

Diagnosis of post-capillary PH

The full diagnostic work-up of systolic and diastolic heart failure is beyond the scope of this book. However, establishing that this is the correct diagnosis is pivotal to any assessment of patients with PH.
- Echocardiography may suggest the diagnosis—PAH is unlikely in the presence of systolic LV dysfunction.
- Severe diastolic dysfunction with significant LA enlargement points toward diastolic dysfunction or restriction.
- Severe aortic or mitral stenosis or regurgitation suggest post-capillary PH, but even moderate abnormalities make a left heart cause a more probable cause of the patient's problem.
- While angina may occur in PAH, it is uncommon except in very advanced disease, and in older patients (age >50 years) ischaemia assessments should be performed.
- Where the wedge is abnormal, confirmation of either pre-capillary or post-capillary PH with direct measurement of LVEDP should be performed as the wedge may be artefactually high or low.
- In the setting of evidence for left heart disease even a normal wedge does not exclude post-capillary PH, especially in dehydrated patients and fluid challenge or exercise assessment may be required.

Treatment of post-capillary PH

- Treatment of the underlying cause is the objective. Systolic heart failure should be managed as per standard algorithms.
- There is no proven treatment for diastolic heart failure. Relief of the cause (usually hypertension) is important.
- Where possible, diuretic therapy is adjusted to normalize LV filling pressures and thus remove the cause of PH.

PH due to chronic lung diseases and/ or hypoxia

26 Lung disease-associated PH   **125**

Lung disease-associated PH

Introduction 126
Diagnostic criteria for IPF (UIP) 127
Clinical features suggestive of ILD 127
Histology of IPF 127
Diagnosing PH in IPF 128
ILD and SSc-PAH 129
Treatment of IPF 129
Treatment of ILD-PH 129
Classification of ILD 129
NSIP 130
Further reading 130

Introduction

- ILD is a group of lung diseases characterized by inflammation and fibrosis, and is one of the conditions in group 3 of the Dana Point classification of PH (PH due to lung diseases and/or hypoxia; see 📖 The Dana Point (2008) clinical classification of PH, p.15).
- Lung biopsy is the gold standard for diagnosis but is performed only occasionally in patients with CTD.
- RFTs and HRCT lung scanning are the main diagnostic methods.
- The most common type of ILD is idiopathic pulmonary fibrosis (IPF; usual interstitial pneumonia [UIP]) (Fig. 26.1). Other types are: hypersensitivity pneumonitis, pulmonary Langerhans cell histiocytosis, asbestosis.
- This chapter focuses on IPF which is associated with CTD and PH and complicates the diagnosis of PAH.

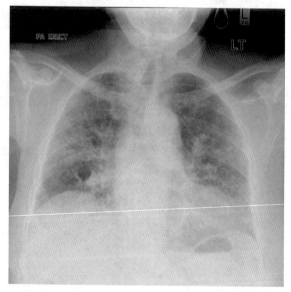

Fig. 26.1 CXR of a patient with pulmonary fibrosis—note extensive reticular and nodular interstitial infiltrate throughout both lung fields with perhaps slight apical sparing. In isolation a CXR lacks sufficient specificity to make a diagnosis.

Diagnostic criteria for IPF (UIP)

Major criteria (all 4 required)

- Exclusion of other known causes of ILD (drugs, exposures, CTDs).
- Abnormal RFTs with evidence of restriction (reduced VC or TLC) and impaired gas exchange (pO_2, $p(A–a)O_2$, DLCO).
- Bibasal reticular abnormalities with minimal ground glass on HRCT scans.
- Transbronchial lung biopsy or bronchoalveolar lavage (BAL) showing no features to support an alternative diagnosis.

Minor criteria (3 of 4 required)

- Age >50.
- Insidious onset of otherwise unexplained exertional dyspnoea.
- Duration of illness >3 months.
- Bibasal inspiratory crackles. PH is common in ILD patients, being present in at least 30% of IPF patients referred for LT reaching over 80% at the time of transplantation. This chapter will focus on PH complicating IPF which is associated with CTD, particularly with the ScL-70 antibody.

Interstitial pneumonias have recently been reclassified into histological conditions. Two of these are IPF or UIP and non-specific interstitial pneumonia (NSIP). IPF/UIP and NSIP are clinically very similar but NSIP, which is associated with SSc, has a far better outcome. However, it remains unclear if NSIP is a truly distinct entity; there is considerable clinical and radiological overlap. The histopathological pattern of NSIP can be found in a wide variety of clinical and radiological contexts.

Clinical features suggestive of ILD

- Patients usually >50 years.
- Insidious onset of otherwise unexplained exertional dyspnoea of ≥6 months' duration, dry cough.
- Bibasal end-inspiratory 'Velcro' crackles, and finger clubbing.
- Bibasal reticular abnormalities on CXR and HRCT scan of the chest (Figs. 26.1 and 26.2).
- Transbronchial lung biopsy or BAL cellular profile with no features to support a specific diagnosis such as sarcoid, pulmonary histiocytosis X, or alveolar proteinosis.

Histology of IPF

There is marked variation in the degree of interstitial fibrosis, inflammation, and fibrotic foci from one area to another, interspersed with adjacent normal pulmonary parenchyma with or without honeycombing but without the presence of granuloma, vasculitis, identifiable infectious agent, or aggregates of lymphocytes or mononuclear cells; and without the characteristic histological features of NSIP, desquamative interstitial pneumonia/respiratory bronchiolitis, acute interstitial pneumonia, eosinophilic pneumonia, or bronchiolitis obliterans organizing pneumonia.

Diagnosing PH in IPF

RHC

- As in other types of PH, RHC is essential for diagnosis. There is no agreed upper limit of mPAP expected in IPF. The mPAP in IPF typicallly ranges between 25–35mmHg.
- No other single test is accurate for diagnosis. A combination of anatomical and physiological tests improves the predictive accuracy in identifying patients who should have RHC.
- Echocardiography is unreliable for diagnosis with a high proportion of false positive and false negative results. Specificity may be as low as 17%. There are often significant technical limitations due to obtaining an adequate echo window.
- There is no correlation between BNP/NTproBNP levels and extent of ILD or lung volumes.

HRCT

There is no correlation between extent of HRCT findings and RHC measurement of mPAP. Ground glass, fibrotic, and honeycombing is similar in ILD patients with and without PH (Fig. 26.2).

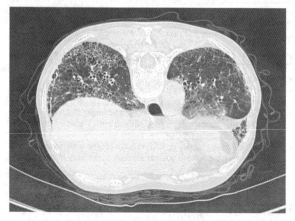

Fig. 26.2 HRCT of a patient with extensive basal pulmonary fibrosis. Note extensive reticular opacities (dominantly subpleural) with some honeycombing and traction bronchiectasis (bronchi that are larger than the accompanying vessels). Extensive parenchymal destruction as observed here can cause elevation of pulmonary pressures simply due to loss of capillary cross-sectional area.

ILD and SSc-PAH

- Diagnosing PAH is often difficult in scleroderma when there is associated ILD.
- An mPAP >35mmHg with a high PVR suggests an SSc pulmonary vasculopathy in addition to ILD-PH.
- DLCO alone is insensitive (sensitivity 50%) for diagnosing PH in ILD patients.
- FVC/DLCO >1.4 identifies 70% of patients with PH.
- A TLC or FVC >70% combined with a DLCO of <60% is helpful in screening for PH.

Treatment of IPF

- There is little evidence from large RCTs that any treatment is effective in reversing lung fibrosis.
- IPF is currently incurable but achieving stability of the disease with preservation of symptoms in some patients is a realistic goal.
- Immunosuppression and anti-inflammatory drugs, using 6, monthly treatments of cyclophosphamide combined with azathioprine, and long-term oral steroids supplemented with steroid-sparing drugs (e.g. myocophenylate) are commonly used treatments.
- The addition of the antioxidant N-acetylcysteine to prednisolone and azathioprine produced a slight benefit in terms of FVC and DLCO over a 12-month follow-up and appeared to be preventive of the myelotoxicity associated with azathioprine.
- Trials of bosentan and of interferon gamma-1b have not shown any benefit.

Treatment of ILD-PH

There is no evidence from prospective, placebo-controlled RCTs that any of the standard PAH treatments (vasodilators, anticoagulants, prostanoids, ERAs), improve survival, or long-term functional capacity or other outcomes. Sildenafil in a small study ↑ 6MWD of 49m after 14 months.

LT may be helpful. For SSc patients in particular, significant oesophageal reflux is a contraindication to LT.

Classification of ILD

ILD is classified into two types histologically and by CT appearances. Lung biopsy is performed in only a small minority of patients.

The former diagnosis of IPF has been reclassified as UIP.

A reticular pattern suggests established interstitial fibrosis and is seen as innumerable interlacing line shadows with associated distortion of the lung architecture. Ground-glass opacification indicates inflammatory infiltration and is seen as a hazy increase in lung parenchymal attenuation, with preservation of bronchial and vascular markings.

NSIP

Most (80%) patients with SSc have NSIP which on CT is characterized by finer fibrosis and a higher proportion of ground-glass opacification and has a better prognosis than UIP which is present in 10% of patients; the remainder have a mixed picture.

The majority of patients with SSc have predominant ground-glass opacification or a mixed pattern, whereas approximately 1/3 of patients had a predominant reticular pattern. There may be traction bronchiectasis but usually no honeycombing which is more typical of UIP.

Further reading

Lettieri CJ, Nathan SD, Barnett SD, et al. Prevalence and outcomes of pulmonary arterial hypertension in advanced idiopathic pulmonary fibrosis. *Chest* 2006; **129**:746–52.

Venous thromboembolism, acute pulmonary embolism, and chronic thromboembolic pulmonary hypertension

27 Venous thromboembolism   **133**

28 Acute pulmonary embolism and investigations   **137**

29 Chronic thromboembolic pulmonary hypertension   **147**

Venous thromboembolism

Introduction *134*
Prevalence of VTE *134*
Risk factors for VTE *134*
Pathophysiology and natural history of VTE *135*
Clinical features of DVT *135*
Outcome after VTE and PE *136*
Investigation of VTE and acute PE *136*
Further reading *136*

Introduction

VTE, including both DVT and acute PE, is common and is the 3rd most common cardiovascular abnormality after acute coronary syndrome and stroke. It may recur, is underdiagnosed, and affects hospitalized and non-hospitalized patients. Long-term complications include fatal and non-fatal PE, CTEPH (up to after 4% of PEs), and post-thrombotic syndrome (PTS), and their associated costs.

VTE results from a combination of hereditary and acquired risk factors, also known as thrombophilia or hypercoagulable states. Over 100 years ago, Rudolf Virchow described the 3 risk factors underlying venous thrombosis:
- Vessel wall damage
- Venous stasis
- ↑ activation of clotting factors.

Prevalence of VTE

The incidence of VTE is unclear because it may be silent or present with sudden death due to PE which may not be documented if a postmortem is not done. In one large postmortem study >1/3 of patients had venous thrombi, including >1/4 having pulmonary emboli.

Risk factors for VTE

- The probability of VTE increases with the greater number of risk factors (Table 27.1).
- Patients with intermediate or high pretest probability of PE require additional diagnostic imaging studies.

Table 27.1 Risk factors for VTE

Hereditary	Acquired
Factor V Leiden mutation	Postoperative: orthopaedic, major abdominal, pelvic surgery
Prothrombin gene mutation	
Protein C or S deficiency	Major trauma and immobility
Antithrombin deficiency	Medical illness and immobility (heart failure, COPD, cancer)
Hyperhomocysteinaemia	
Elevated levels of factor VIII	Pregnancy, oral contraceptives, hormone replacement therapy
Dysfibrinogenaemia	
	Indwelling central venous catheters or pacemaker electrodes and local thrombosis
	Cancer or certain cancer treatments
	APS
	Heparin-induced thrombocytopenia
	Inflammatory bowel disease
	Myeloproliferative disorders
	Air travel, immobility and venous stagnation
	Body mass index >30
	Previous VTE

Pathophysiology and natural history of VTE

Venous thrombi, composed of red blood cells, platelets, and leukocytes bound together by fibrin, form in sites of vessel damage and areas of stagnant blood flow such as the valve pockets of the deep veins of the calf or thigh. Thrombi either remain in the peripheral veins, where they eventually undergo endogenous fibrinolysis and recanalization, or they embolize to the PAs and cause PE.

DVT

The leg veins are the most common site for DVT. 50% of untreated proximal leg DVTs (popliteal vein and above) result in PEs. Without treatment, approximately 25% of calf vein thrombi propagate to involve the popliteal vein or migrate to a more proximal vein.

Pathophysiology and consequences of PE

- Impairment of gas exchange due to impaired perfusion but not ventilation.
- Intrapulmonary shunting leading to hypoxaemia.
- Atelectasis and vasoconstriction resulting from the release of inflammatory mediators (serotonin and thromboxane).
- Major proximal PEs cause acute increases in PVR, leading to RV impairment and a fall in CO and BP. Collapse and death may occur and are more likely in patients with coronary heart disease and pre-existing heart failure.
- Angina and right heart failure may occur due to ↑ RV wall tension, ↑ RVEDP, and ↓ flow in the right coronary artery.

Clinical features of DVT

- Pain and tenderness.
- Erythema and the presence of dilated veins (collaterals) on the leg (or chest wall in arm DVT).
- Swelling and oedema.
- Increased warmth.

The clinical diagnosis of DVT is unreliable. Clinical probability scores based on clinical features and risk factors may aid risk stratification (see Table 27.1). The negative predictive value for DVT in low probability patients is 96%. Imaging in low probability patients is usually not necessary. High probability patients have a positive predictive value of <75% and may need further tests.

Outcome after VTE and PE

• Post-thrombotic syndrome occurs in 30% of patients within a few years after DVT; 25% of these may develop a chronic venous stasis ulcer.
• Mortality rate for untreated PE treatment is >30% and 2–8% with adequate therapy.
• 4% of PE patients develop CTEPH within 2 years of PE.

Investigation of VTE and acute PE

D-dimer testing

A low pretest probability plus a negative D-dimer has a high negative predictive value for VTE (>99%).

A positive D dimer does not confirm the diagnosis of DVT. False-positive results are seen in patients with malignancy, trauma, recent surgery, infection, pregnancy, and active bleeding.

Duplex ultrasonography (DU)

DU is the imaging procedure of choice for the diagnosis of DVT because it is readily available and is less invasive and less costly than other procedures. It has a sensitivity and specificity of about 95% and 98%, respectively, for detecting DVT in symptomatic patients. It is operator dependent and less sensitive in asymptomatic patients and for detecting calf vein thrombi. DU cannot always distinguish between acute and chronic DVT and may be difficult to perform on obese patients. An inability to compress the vein with the ultrasound transducer is considered diagnostic for DVT. Other findings that are suggestive but not diagnostic include venous distention, absent or ↓ spontaneous flow, and abnormal Doppler signals. In patients with a low pretest probability of DVT or PE, a negative high-sensitivity D-dimer indicates a low likelihood of VTE.

Contrast venography

Contrast venography has been the gold standard test for the diagnosis of DVT. The presence of an intraluminal filling defect is diagnostic, although abrupt cut-offs, non-filling of the deep venous system, or demonstration of collateral flow may raise suspicion for the presence of DVT. Venography is invasive and requires the use of potentially harmful contrast agents; therefore, it has largely been replaced by non-invasive tests.

Other diagnostic tests

Less frequently used tests to detect DVT include magnetic resonance venography imaging (MRV) and computed axial tomography venography. Their place has yet to be defined.

Further reading

Huisman MV, Klok FA. Diagnostic management of clinically suspected acute pulmonary embolism. *J Thromb Haemost* 2009; **7**(Suppl 1):312–17.
Squizzato A, Galli M, Dentali F, et al. Outpatient treatment and early discharge of symptomatic pulmonary embolism: a systematic review. *Eur Respir J* 2009; **33**(5):1148–55.

Acute pulmonary embolism and investigations

Clinical features of acute PE *138*
Clinical decision rules *138*
Imaging for suspected acute PE *140*
Treatment of DVT *141*
Treatment of acute PE *142*
Prevention and screening *144*
DVT of the arm *144*
Phlegmasia cerulea dolens *145*
Pregnancy and VTE *145*
Further reading *145*

Clinical features of acute PE

- Pleuritic chest pain and breathlessness.
- Apprehension, cough, haemoptysis, syncope.
- Tachycardia, added heart sounds.
- Signs of right heart failure.

Clinical decision rules

Pretest probability scores or clinical decision rules also have a role in the diagnosis of acute PE. The absence of risk factors or signs of a DVT, with at least a medium probability of another explanation, indicates a very low probability of PE (see Box 28.1).

Only 0.5% of patients with a low probability of PE and a negative D dimmer would develop VTE.

> **Box 28.1** Features increasing probability for PE
> - Clinical signs and symptoms of DVT (leg swelling and pain of the deep leg veins).
> - Features of PE (breathlessness, pleuritic chest pain, rub, tachypnoea).
> - Alternative diagnosis less likely than PE.
> - HR >100bpm.
> - Immobilization (>3 days) or surgery in the previous week.
> - Previous PE or DVT.
> - Haemoptysis.
> - Malignancy (receiving treatment or treated in last 6 months or palliative).

ECG

The ECG has a low positive and low negative predictive accuracy for PE. Signs of PE depend on the extent of pulmonary infarction and PH.
- $S_1Q_3T_3$ has a low sensitivity and specificity
- Non-specific findings include sinus tachycardia, atrial fibrillation (AF), and right bundle branch block.

CXR

A normal CXR helps exclude other causes of breathlessness, e.g. pneumonia and infections with consolidation, malignancy and pleural effusion, interstitial lung disease and pneumothorax.

Signs of PE include pleural effusion and consolidation.

Arterial blood gas analysis

- A normal PaO_2 does not rule out PE.
- Hypoxia (<80mmHg) in the absence of cardiovascular and lung disease increases the probability of PE. In the Prospective Investigation of Pulmonary Embolism Diagnosis (PIOPED) study, only 26% of patients with angiographically proven PE had a PaO_2 >80mmHg.

- In patients with cardiopulmonary collapse, a normal PaO_2 suggests an alternative diagnosis. Similarly, an elevated alveolar–arterial gradient is suggestive but not specific for the diagnosis of an acute PE. Therefore if the alveolar–arterial gradient is normal, an acute PE cannot be excluded.

Biomarkers (troponins and brain natriuretic peptide)

Elevated levels of cardiac troponins correlate with echocardiographic findings of RVP overload in patients with acute PE and overall mortality. In-hospital complications are higher in patients with elevated troponin compared to those with normal levels. Brain natriuretic peptide (BNP) elevation in the absence of renal dysfunction is also a marker of RV dysfunction in patients with PE and has also been shown to predict adverse outcome in patients with acute PE.

Echocardiography (transthoracic and transoesophageal)

- >50% of haemodynamically stable patients with PE do not have evidence of RV dysfunction on transthoracic echocardiography (TTE).
- Patients with haemodynamic collapse may have severe RV dysfunction, RV dilatation, and a raised TVR suggesting PH.
- TTE or transoesophageal echocardiography (TOE) is useful for bedside evaluation in the ITU or CCU. Findings of PE and PH include: RV dilatation, RV hypokinesis, tricuspid regurgitation, septal flattening, paradoxical septal motion, diastolic LV impairment secondary to septal displacement, lack of inspiratory collapse of the inferior vena cava (IVC), and occasionally direct visualization of the thrombus.

See also Chapter 14.

Imaging for suspected acute PE

Ventilation perfusion scanning

- Nuclear medicine scans are extremely accurate in excluding PEs. Scans showing normal ventilation and perfusion virtually exclude PE. However, mis-matched or matched defects are common in many conditions other than PE.
- A positive diagnosis on nuclear screening can be made only in the setting of normal chest radiology.
- Multiple perfusion defects in the absence of ventilation defects, in a patient with a normal CXR indicate a high probability of acute PE.
- Most patients with suspected PEs have pulmonary comorbidities, and so definitive results are not uncommon.

CTPA

Iodine contrast CT, timed to image the chest when contrast opacifies the PAs, is now the most common method of diagnosing PEs (Fig. 28.1).

- The use of contrast agents in sick patients may cause renal impairment, especially if the patient is not adequately hydrated.
- In acute PE, filling defects are confined to intraluminal clot and occluded or missing vessels; additional information is obtained from lung windows showing areas of hypoperfusion.
- A negative CTPA is extremely accurate provided consideration is given to the presence of all major branches and the absence of perfusion defects. However, not all radiologists are trained to report in this fashion.
- Some additional information can be gleaned from observing the right heart on CTPA, which is distended in severe PE; relative underfilling of the LV may also be evident.

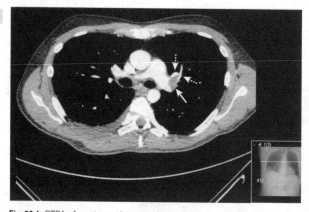

Fig. 28.1 CTPA of a patient with acute pulmonary embolism. Note semi-occlusive contrast defect within the left main pulmonary artery (solid arrow), contrast skirting around the edges (dashed arrows) confirm that this is truly intraluminal and not yet adherent to the walls.

Treatment of DVT

It is helpful to discuss complex cases of known or suspected DVT with a vascular surgeon and/or radiologist.

Treatment for DVT includes prevention of PE and PTS, and recurrent thrombosis. Once DVT is suspected, anticoagulation should be started immediately unless there is a contraindication.

Anticoagulation for DVT and PE

Low-molecular-weight heparin (LMWH)

LMWH is preferred for the initial inpatient treatment of DVT. Either unfractionated heparin (UFH) or LMWH is acceptable for PE. Outpatient treatment of DVT with LMWH is safe and cost-effective for carefully selected patients. LMWH is safe and efficacious for the long-term treatment of VTE in select individuals and may be preferable for cancer patients.

- Enoxaparin is given either as a once-daily injection (1.5mg/kg/day) or twice per day (1mg/kg every 12h) and two other agents are available, dalteparin and tinzaparin. No monitoring is required except in renal insufficiency or in obese, paediatric, or pregnant patients.
- LMWH is generally avoided in severe renal impairment as renal excretion is reduced and can result in bleeding complications.

Unfractionated heparin (UFH)

UFH can also be given using an IV loading dose of 80U/kg bolus followed by 18U/kg/h IV continuous infusion or by intermittent subcutaneous injection. Intermittent IV injection of UFH is no longer recommended. An oral anticoagulant (usually warfarin), is started at the same time as heparin or a factor Xa inhibitor is started. Heparin, with daily monitoring of the APTT, is continued usually for 5 days until the INR is stable at a therapeutic level for 2 consecutive days.

VTE during pregnancy

Heparins, and not warfarin, are used for the management of VTE in pregnancy because heparin and LMWH do not cross the placenta. LMWH are preferred to UFH because they have a lower risk of osteoporosis and of heparin-induced thrombocytopenia.

Factor Xa inhibitors

Fondaparinux is an indirect factor Xa inhibitor that can be used as VTE prophylaxis, treatment of DVT and PE, and for acute coronary syndromes. It should be used with caution in renal impairment and is contraindicated in patients with severe renal impairment (creatinine clearance <30mL/min) and bacterial endocarditis.

Thrombolytic therapy for DVT

Thrombolytics, preferably given by local infusion into the affected vein, may be beneficial in patients who have extensive proximal DVT and a low risk of bleeding. Although it has been suggested that use of thrombolytics promotes early recanalization and minimizes the incidence of the PTS, their role in the treatment of DVT without a threatened limb is still unclear.

Treatment of acute PE

Anticoagulation and thrombolysis for PE

For known or moderately high-risk PE, UFH, LMWH, or fondaparinux should be started immediately.

- Echocardiography and measurement of NTpro BNP help evaluate the effects of PE on the RV. If the patient is normotensive and the RV size and function are normal, standard anticoagulation is advised.
- Thrombolysis should be considered for normotensive patients with dilatation of the RV. Thrombolysis and pulmonary embolectomy should be considered for hypotensive patients but this is controversial because no clear short-term mortality benefit has been shown, and the risk of pulmonary embolectomy is >20%.
- In haemodynamically unstable patients, tissue plasminogen activator (rtPA) given as a 100mg infusion over 2h may be given. Bleeding remains the most serious complication of thrombolytic therapy. Local administration of these agents via catheter-directed therapy is not recommended due to the risk of haemorrhage at the insertion site. The risk of intracranial bleeding is 1–2%.

Pulmonary embolectomy

Although there is no evidence from RCTs, pulmonary embolectomy is rarely used to treat haemodynamically compromised PE despite heparin and failed thrombolysis, or when thrombolysis is contraindicated. The role of catheter-based embolectomy procedures that use aspiration, fragmentation, or rheolytic therapy are experimental.

Vena caval interruption

Routine use of IVC filters for the treatment of VTE is not recommended.

Indications for IVC in selected patients include:
- Contraindication to anticoagulation.
- Complications of anticoagulation.
- Recurrent thromboembolism despite adequate anticoagulant therapy.
- Patients undergoing pulmonary endarterectomy.

Relative indications for IVC filters are:
- Massive PE.
- Iliocaval DVT.
- Free-floating proximal DVT.
- Cardiac or pulmonary insufficiency.
- High risk of complications from anticoagulation (frequent falls, ataxia).
- Poor compliance.

Retrievable filters may be considered when anticoagulation is temporarily contraindicated or there is a short duration of PE risk. The indications for placing a retrievable IVC filter are the same as for permanent devices. IVC filter alone is not effective therapy for DVT and resumption of anticoagulation as soon as possible after placement is recommended.

New anticoagulants

Argatroban (Argatroban®), bivalirudin (Angiomax®), and lepirudin (Refludan®) are direct thrombin inhibitors approved for treatment of heparin-induced thrombocytopenia (HIT). None, however, is currently licensed for VTE.

- Of the newer oral drugs, direct factor Xa inhibitors rivaroxaban and the direct thrombin inhibitor dabigatran etexilate are approved in the EU for the prevention of VTE in adult patients undergoing elective total hip- or knee-replacement surgery.
- Dabigatran was more effective than warfarin in reducing the risk of stroke in patients with AF, and the risk of bleeding is lower (RE-LY study). There is a low risk of drug or food interactions, and no need for routine monitoring of the INR but it should be used cautiously in patients with renal impairment. It is considerably more expensive than warfarin.
- The impact of the new agents will be influenced by the balance between efficacy and safety, improved convenience for patient and physician, and any potential cost-effectiveness benefits.

Warfarin

Warfarin is the drug of first choice for long-term treatment of VTE, maintaining an INR of 2–3 and in high risk cases, 2.5–3.5. Treatment for first DVT due to a transient cause in a patient at low risk from further VTE is 3 months. If the risk is at least moderate, then anticoagulation should be for 6 months. Duration depends on a patient's individual risk of recurrent thrombosis vs risk of bleeding (see Box 28.2).

Box 28.2 Risk factors for recurrence of VTE
- ♂ gender.
- Increasing age.
- ↑ body mass index.
- Neurologic disease (with extremity paresis).
- Malignancy.
- APS.
- Idiopathic VTE.
- Strong family history of VTE.
- Antithrombin, protein C and S deficiencies.
- Homozygous for Factor V Leiden.
- Doubly heterozygous for Factor V Leiden and prothrombin gene mutation.
- Elevated D-dimer following discontinuation of warfarin.
- Persistent residual DVT.
- Permanent IVC filter.

Long-term anticoagulation is recommended for prophylaxis against VTE in patients who have:
- APS.
- Homozygous for Factor V Leiden, or doubly heterozygous for Factor V Leiden and prothrombin gene mutation.
- Active malignancy and 'unexplained' recurrent DVTs.
- Patients with CTEPH.

Compression stockings and PTS

Thrombotic damage to the venous valves can lead to venous hypertension and PTS with an incidence of 30% at 8 years.

Clinical features of PTS
- Oedema.
- Skin changes (↑ pigmentation and lipodermatosclerosis).
- Pain.
- Venous stasis ulceration in severe cases.

Incidence of PTS is reduced with the use of compression stockings. They are used at a compression pressure of 30–40mmHg for 1–2 years following an acute DVT.

Prevention and screening

Prevention

PE remains the most common preventable cause of hospital death in developed countries. The majority of VTEs occur in hospital and many of these could be prevented with adequate prophylaxis.

Without prophylaxis, the incidence of hospital-acquired DVT is 10–20% among medical patients and even higher (15–40%) among surgical patients. Adequate prophylaxis reduces the incidence with a 62% reduction in fatal PE, 57% reduction in non-fatal PE, and 53% reduction in DVT.

Screening for DVT

Screening asymptomatic patients for DVT is labour intensive and cost ineffective. Thus, prophylaxis in at-risk populations remains the most effective means for preventing complications of VTE.

DVT of the arm

This is usually due to thrombosis in or around a central venous catheter, pacemaker electrode or infection and thrombosis related to IV drug abuse, and less commonly to thoracic outlet syndrome (also referred to as effort thrombosis) and hypercoagulable conditions including malignancy. Patients may be asymptomatic or complain of arm swelling and pain. It may be necessary to remove the focus of thrombosis. Anticoagulation is indicated if there are no contraindications. Thrombolysis should be considered in cases of acute or recent onset.

Phlegmasia cerulea dolens

Phlegmasia cerulea dolens (gross swelling and reduced perfusion of a limb due to venous obstruction) is a vascular emergency requiring anticoagulation or, in select cases, thrombolysis or surgical or catheter-based thrombectomy. Fasciotomy may also be required to relieve associated compartment syndromes.

Pregnancy and VTE

VTE is the leading cause of maternal death. The risk of VTE during pregnancy is ↑ 4-fold; this risk is ↑ 5-fold for 6 weeks following delivery.

Risks for VTE during pregnancy include:
- Age >35 years.
- Caesarean section.
- Pre-eclampsia.
- A history of previous VTE or family history of thrombosis.

Further reading

Cash C, Cleverley J. Imaging in acute and chronic pulmonary thromboembolic disease. In: D Abraham, C Handler, M Dashwood, et al. (eds) *Advances in Vascular Medicine*, pp. 247–72. London: Springer; 2010.

Chronic thromboembolic pulmonary hypertension

Introduction 148
Anticoagulation 148
Medical treatment for inoperable CTEPH 148
Pulmonary endarterectomy 149
Indications for PEA 150
Surgical technique 150
Haemodynamic changes after PEA 150
Perioperative mortality 150
Functional class after PEA 150
Survival in CTEPH 150
Further reading 151

Introduction

- 1–3.8% of patients with acute PEs may develop CTEPH.
- Only 1/3 of patients with confirmed CTED have a history of acute PE and so a history negative for PEs is unreliable in excluding the possibility of CTEPH.
- PEs may be the main cause of PH but other heart and lung conditions may coexist and contribute to breathlessness and PH.
- 1/3 patients are found to have thrombophilia on investigation, 3.5% have a history of splenectomy and such patients are more likely to have inoperable disease.
- CTEPH is potentially surgically treatable and so it is important that PEs are considered in all patients with PH.
- 2/3 of patients with CTEPH are operable; all patients should be considered for operation by an expert in CTEPH surgery.

Anticoagulation

This is the most important aspect of treatment and should be continued for life with a tightly controlled INR of 2.0–3.0 to prevent further thromboembolism.

- CTEPH cannot be diagnosed until 3 months of anticoagulation has failed to resolve the obstructions.
- LMWH is used in patients who cannot take warfarin. There is no evidence yet that new forms of antithrombotic agents are superior to warfarin.
- The direct thrombin inhibitor, dabigatran etexilate, and other new anticoagulants, including the oral factor Xa inhibitors, rivaroxaban, apixaban, and edoxaban, the parenteral factor Xa inhibitor, idrabiotaparinux, and the novel VKA, tecarfarin, are currently being assessed in other thrombotic conditions. Dabigatran has been shown to be safer than warfarin in AF.
- In patients with a thrombotic tendency or lupus anticoagulant antibodies, and following pulmonary endarterectomy (PEA), the INR is maintained between 2.5–3.5.
- Anticoagulation should not be stopped unless there are important reasons. Patients are switched to self-administered subcutaneous clexane if warfarin is stopped for cardiac catheterization or other reasons.

Medical treatment for inoperable CTEPH

- There are no data from long-term RCTs that any PAH targeted therapy alone or in combination improves mortality, symptoms, or functional capacity. Only small, short-term studies have been performed. The majority of studies have been uncontrolled.
- Registry data shows a much improved survival in inoperable CTEPH patients associated with the use of pulmonary vasodilator therapy.

- Bosentan has been shown to improve haemodynamics over 16 weeks but no improvement in 6MWD.
- Medical treatment is used in patients not suitable for PEA due to distal disease, or because of significant comorbidity which would make PEA prohibitively risky, or severe RV impairment which would ↑ the perioperative risk, and in those with recurrent VTE or persistent PH after PEA.
- It is not clear whether combination therapy is more effective than monotherapy in any form of CTEPH either in non-operable patients or those after PEA. Patients may also receive non-targeted therapy with diuretics and digoxin.
- ERAs and/or sildenafil are used in patients who are in WHO class III.
- Prostacyclins are used for patients in WHO class IV and also in an attempt to improve haemodynamics prior to PEA ('bridging therapy').
- Medical treatment of right heart failure may require diuretics to alleviate peripheral oedema, and digoxin may also be used, although again, there is no evidence base for this in CTEPH.

Pulmonary endarterectomy

This is the preferred treatment for CTEPH. Papworth Hospital (Cambridge) is currently the only UK hospital offering this service. The diagnosis of CTEPH must be secure and other causes of PH excluded because PEA offers the potential of a cure.

- In-hospital survival >95%, and 1-year survival >90%.
- >1/10 have major sequelae including neurological complications.
- PAP falls dramatically in most patients, though normal levels (mPAP <20mmHg are uncommon).
- Significant residual PH is seen in 17%; adverse medium-term outcomes are seen mainly in this subgroup.
- Most symptomatic patients with at least 5 segmental vessels diseased or occluded (25% of the total) and a PVR of <1000 dynes.s.cm^{-5} get a good result from surgery and are at low risk (<2%) from complications.
- Patients with a very high PVR (>1000 dynes.s.cm^{-5}) 'out of proportion' to visible thrombus and obstruction to blood flow, a mPAP >50mmHg, cardiac index (CI) <2.0, and WHO class IV, identify high-risk patients and suggest inoperable small vessel arteriopathy and a separate pathology of PAH. Surgery is less likely to be successful in this group. The operative mortality is 20% in patients with a PVR >1200 dynes.s.cm.$^{-5}$. The higher the PASP the higher the mortality but suprasystemic PAP is not a contraindication to PEA.
- It is, however, only at operation when the ease of dissection and the ability to clear obstructive material, can this decision be made with certainty. A lot depends on the experience of the surgeon reviewing the data with colleagues at a multidisciplinary meeting.

There are no accepted guidelines identifying those patients who should be treated with disease-modifying drugs post PEA, but >15% of patients, mainly those with persistently high mPAPs and those with less than optimum surgical results, are treated post PEA.

Indications for PEA

The surgeon makes a decision whether PEA would result in worthwhile clearance from the PAs. Echocardiography, 6MWT, full lung function tests, RHC, and CTPA, invasive pulmonary angiography, or MRPA. Patients aged >50 years also have coronary angiography and carotid Doppler testing.

An IVC filter is inserted before surgery although there is no evidence base for this.

Surgical technique

The aim is to perform a full endarterectomy (not thrombectomy or embolectomy) of both pulmonary vascular trees. Access is via a median sternotomy with hypothermic cardiopulmonary bypass and right and left pulmonary arteriotomies within the pericardium. The patient is cooled to 20°C.

Haemodynamic changes after PEA

Both mPAP and PVR fall significantly (reported mPAP 52mmHg to 23mmHg; PVR 744 to 217 dynes.cm.s^{-5}) on the first postoperative day, but these changes may be influenced by several factors unrelated to PEA.

Perioperative mortality

In-hospital mortality from PEA in carefully selected patients is <5%.

Functional class after PEA

6MWD increases from 276±17m to 375±14m 3 months after PEA and further to 394±15m at 1 year.

Survival in CTEPH

The 3-year survival before the availability of modern treatments was 10%. 1- and 3-year survivals rates for medically treated patients with inoperable CTEPH with targeted therapies are 83% and 76% respectively. In one study using Bosentan for non-surgically suitable disease and for persistent PH post PEA, 1-year survival was 96%. Recurrent PEs are unlikely with effective anticoagulation.

Further reading

Jenkins DP. Surgical management of chronic thromboembolic pulmonary hypertension (CTEPH). D Abraham, C Handler, M Dashwood, *et al.* (eds) *Advances in Vascular Medicine*, pp. 233–46. London: Springer; 2010.

Pepke-Zaba J. Chronic thromboembolic pulmonary hypertension. In: D Abraham, C Handler, M Dashwood, *et al.* (eds) *Advances in Vascular Medicine*, pp. 215–24. London: Springer; 2010.

Suntharalingam J, Morrell NW. Pathophysiology of chronic thromboembolic pulmonary hypertension (CTEPH). In: D Abraham, C Handler, M Dashwood, *et al.* (eds) *Advances in Vascular Medicine*, pp. 225–31. London: Springer; 2010.

Diagnosis and investigations in PAH

30 Diagnosis and investigations in PAH   **155**

Diagnosis and investigations in PAH

General principles of diagnostic approach 156
Diagnostic algorithm 159
Simple investigations 161
V/Q scanning 164
High resolution computed tomography 166
Pulmonary angiography and magnetic resonance scanning 167
Cardiac magnetic resonance imaging (CMR) 171
Echocardiography 173
Echocardiographic assessment of the RV 176
Non-invasive exercise testing 184
Cardiac catheterization 186
Acute vasodilator testing 194

General principles of diagnostic approach

Progressive thickening and narrowing of the small (<0.5mm) PAs due to proliferation, fibrosis, and vasoconstriction lead to an increase in PVR and pressure overload on the RV. This leads to RV hypertrophy, dilatation, and ultimately RV failure and death. When the RV fails, the prognosis is poor. Markers of a poor prognosis reflect RV failure.

Prognostic markers of RV failure and death

- Poor functional capacity (New York Heart Association class, and reduced 6MWD).
- Rapid progression of symptoms.
- Falling saturations and/or BP on exercise.
- High mRAP.
- Reduced CI.
- Progressive increase in NTproBNP.
- RA dilatation, reduced TAPSE, or LV compression on echocardiography.

RV function can recover after successful LT or thromboendarterectomy for CTEPH.

Symptoms of PAH

The average delay between onset of symptoms to diagnosis is >2 years. This delays treatment. PAH is often advanced by the time of diagnosis with 75% of patients in WHO classes III or IV. Symptoms occur only after there has been extensive pulmonary vascular obliteration. The pathological and haemodynamic changes are usually well established before a diagnosis is made.

This underlines the importance of screening in high-risk groups (SSc, HIV, POPH).

This delay is due to the
- Lack of awareness of the condition by both clinicians and patients (compared with acute MI or chronic lung diseases).
- Lack of symptoms until the condition is quite advanced, particularly in young patients with a compliant RV.
- The vague, non-specific symptoms of PAH (breathlessness, tiredness, fatigue, leading to a misdiagnosis of 'out of shape or unfit, depressed').
- The lack of a simple non-invasive 'rule in' or 'rule out' test.
- When symptoms occur, they are ascribed to a more common cardio-respiratory disease, e.g. asthma.

PAH should be considered in all patients with unexplained breathlessness.

Irrespective of the type of PAH and any associated condition, the most common symptom is gradually progressive shortness of breath noticed when patients exert themselves walking up hills or stairs, or doing gardening or housework. Fatigue and weakness are common. Feeling lightheaded during exercise and exertional syncope indicate severe PAH. Ankle swelling, nausea, and abdominal swelling reflect right heart failure.

Patients with CTD-PAH may believe these symptoms are simply part of their underlying CTD. Screening programmes for PAH in this important and sizeable 'at risk subgroup' is aimed to detect PAH early.

Only a minority, 4%, of patients with PE develop CTEPH. Most at risk are those with massive PE and/or previous thromboembolism. Most but not all patients with CTEPH give a history of PE which may be clinically silent. CTEPH may occur without PE due to thrombotic and/or inflammatory processes in the PAs.

> Breathless patients with a history of VTE should have echocardiography and if necessary, CTPA.

WHO functional classification of PAH

Patients with PAH are classified into the following WHO classes:
- *I*. No limitation of usual physical activity.
- *II*. Slight limitation of physical activity with ordinary activities but comfortable at rest. More than ordinary exertion causes breathlessness, fatigue, chest pain, or syncope.
- *III*. Marked limitation of physical activity with even slight exertion but comfortable at rest.
- *IV*. Patients are breathless and/or fatigued at rest and cannot carry out any physical activity without symptoms. They may have signs of right heart failure

Signs of PAH

These depend on the severity of PAH, the presence of right heart failure, the underlying condition, the age of the patient, and their ability to tolerate the increase in PAP.
- In early PAH the examination is often normal.
- The first physical signs include a left parasternal lift, and a loud P2 which may be palpable.
- As the PAP and PVR increase putting a pressure load on the RV resulting in heart failure, tachycardia, tachypnoea, cyanosis, raised venous pressure, murmur of tricuspid regurgitation, RV 3rd sound, an enlarged liver with oedema (may not be present in SSc due to tightness of the skin), may be present and should be looked for.
- Lung sounds are usually normal, though effusions reduce basal sounds and may lead to bronchial breathing due to compression. Crepitations, suggest that secondary causes such as lung fibrosis or heart failure may be present.
- Crackles may also be present in PVOD.

Signs of associated disease

- Signs of SSc include induration of the subcutaneous tissue and tightening of the skin of the hands and feet (LSSc) and less commonly, the whole body (DSSc). Telangiectasia, microstomia, calcinosis, loss of finger pulp, autoamputation of fingers and toes.
- Signs of other CTDs such as lupus, dermatomyositis, polymyositis, or Sjögren's syndrome
- Signs of chronic liver disease: finger clubbing, spider naevi, palmar erythema, signs of portal hypertension, may be present in portopulmonary hypertension.
- Signs of HIV: if untreated, lymphadenopathy, candidiasis, Kaposi's sarcoma, signs of opportunistic infection.
- The signs in CTEPH are similar to other causes of PH but there may also be pulmonary flow murmurs heard best with the patient holding their breath in mid-inspiration. There may also be signs of previous DVT.

6MWT

This is a useful test of functional capacity and is used to aid prognostic stratification, and monitor the progression of disease and its response to treatment. Guidelines are published by the American Thoracic Society. The corridor should be long enough (20–40m) without obstacles (in clinic, these are most usually other patients) and patients should not be 'encouraged' during the test. The arterial oxygen saturations are tested both before and after the test, and the BORG score (self-perceived level of discomfort during the test), at the end of the test.

The 6MWT has limitations in certain patients and patient groups including elderly patients and those with musculoskeletal problems (CTD).

Diagnostic algorithm

PAH may be suspected clinically or from non-invasive testing (echocardiography or lung function tests) in patients at risk. A diagnosis of PH due to left heart lung diseases, CTEPH, or PAH is made by other tests. Characterization of PAH and any associated cause is done with blood tests, genetic tests, and imaging. The order of tests is tailored to the clinical situation. See Fig. 30.1.

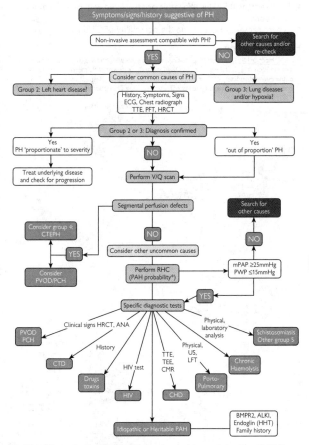

Fig. 30.1 Diagnostic algorithm for PH. Reprinted with permission from Guidelines for the diagnosis and treatment of pulmonary hypertension. *Eur Heart J* 2009; **30**:2493–537. Published by OUP (see Further Reading p 160).

Diagnostic tests for PAH

Because of the complexity of associated conditions with PAH, it is very helpful to have the advice of a multispecialty group of cardiologists, respiratory physicians, rheumatologists, haematologists, and specialists in HIV, infectious diseases, and CHD to evaluate the different test results.

The roles of diagnostic tests are 4-fold:
* To establish whether PH is present (mPAP ≥25mmHg).
* To exclude non-PAH causes of PH.
* To determine if PAH is idiopathic or associated with other relevant conditions.
* Where present to determine the operability of CTEPH.

Further reading

Galiè N, Hoeper MM, Humbert M, *et al.* Guidelines for the diagnosis and treatment of pulmonary hypertension. The Task Force for the Diagnosis and Treatment of Pulmonary Hypertension of the European Society of Cardiology (ESC) and the European Respiratory Society (ERS), endorsed by the International Society of Heart and Lung Transplantation (ISHLT). *Eur Heart J* 2009; **30**:2493–537.

Simple investigations

ECG

This has a low sensitivity (55%) and specificity (70%) in diagnosing and excluding PAH, and therefore is not recommended to screen for PAH, though it is an important part of the diagnostic work-up.

- In advanced PAH with RV hypertrophy there may be tachycardia, large P waves due to RA dilatation, RV hypertrophy with right bundle branch block, and right axis deviation.
- Atrial and/ventricular ectopic beats may be seen in PAH but these are also part of normality and non-specific.
- AF and supraventricular arrhythmias resulting in palpitation are more common in patients with atrial enlargement. Serious ventricular arrhythmias appear to be rare. Heart block is no more common in PAH compared to those without PAH.
- AF has a major impact in PAH, reducing CO with ↑ breathlessness and heart failure. It should be investigated and ideally sinus rhythm restored in order to optimize haemodynamics.
- In post-capillary PH due to LV impairment there may be Q waves from previous infarction, LV hypertrophy due to hypertension, ST-T wave abnormalities due to ischaemia, hypertension, or may be non-specific, and left bundle branch block due to cardiomyopathy or previous infarction.

CXR

A normal CXR does not exclude PH.

The following features help in diagnosis:

- The majority of patients with symptomatic IPAH have an abnormal CXR, showing central PA dilatation. On a PA film a transverse diameter of the right descending PA >16mm suggests PH. Pruning or loss of the peripheral blood vessels.
- An enlarged heart due to LV hypertrophy and dilatation with pulmonary venous hypertension and pulmonary oedema indicate left heart disease and possible PH.
- Hyperinflation (emphysema).
- Lung fibrosis (consider SSc if present) (Fig. 26.1).
- The RV can be reliably seen only on a lateral CXR and may be enlarged in severe PH.
- The CXR may be unremarkable in CTEPH:
- A normal CXR does not exclude PE. If the CXR is normal, the chances of obtaining a diagnostic V/Q scan increase and it is usually the next investigation.
- Westermark's sign of ↑ transradiancy of the affected lung due to pulmonary oligaemia is rarely if ever seen and more likely to be due to technical factors in obtaining a CXR in the acute setting.
- 'Hampton's hump' describes an area of infarct seen as a wedge-shaped opacity adjacent to the visceral pleural space with its convex apex directed to the hilum and although rare, is a useful clue to the diagnosis. Fig. 30.2 shows the typical chest radiography appearance of advanced PAH, with relatively normal lungs, a dilated heart, and grossly enlarged PAs.
- Pleural effusions where present are a sign of heart failure (right or left).

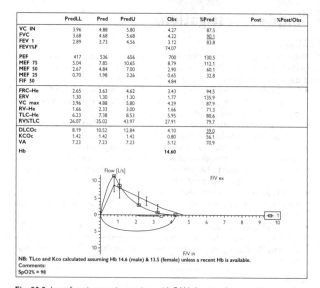

	PredLL	Pred	PredU	Obs	%Pred	Post	%Post/Obs
VC IN	3.96	4.88	5.80	4.27	87.5		
FVC	3.68	4.68	5.68	4.22	90.1		
FEV 1	2.89	3.73	4.56	3.12	83.8		
FEV1%F				74.07			
PEF	417	536	656	700	130.5		
MEF 75	5.04	7.85	10.65	8.79	112.1		
MEF 50	2.67	4.84	7.00	2.90	60.1		
MEF 25	0.70	1.98	3.26	0.65	32.8		
FIF 50				4.84			
FRC–He	2.65	3.63	4.62	3.43	94.5		
ERV	1.30	1.30	1.30	1.77	135.9		
VC max	3.96	4.88	5.80	4.29	87.9		
RV–He	1.66	2.33	3.00	1.66	71.3		
TLC–He	6.23	7.38	8.53	5.95	80.6		
RV%TLC	26.07	35.02	43.97	27.91	79.7		
DLCOc	8.19	10.52	12.84	4.10	39.0		
KCOc	1.42	1.42	1.42	0.80	56.1		
VA	7.23	7.23	7.23	5.12	70.9		
Hb				14.60			

NB: TLco and Kco calculated assuming Hb 14.6 (male) & 13.5 (female) unless a recent Hb is available.
Comments:
SpO2% = 98

Fig. 30.2 Lung function test in a patient with PAH showing disproportionate reduction in DLCO to 39% of predicted compared to the TLC (81% of predicted) and FVC (90% of predicted).

Lung function tests

These help identify the presence and significance of obstructive and/or restrictive lung conditions, and lung fibrosis. Obstructive ventilatory defects suggest non-associated obstructive lung disease from smoking.

> Importantly in PAH the lung function changes are very modest when compared to the symptomatic limitation. Recognition of this discrepancy is vital to ensuring patients are not labelled as having asthma or COPD.

Normal lung function does not exclude PAH.

- Serial changes in lung function test results are helpful in diagnosis, management, and assessing progression of disease. In ILD, progressive lung fibrosis results in progressive matched decline in DLCO and TLC.
- In PAH there may be a mild (60–80% of predicted) disproportionate decrease in DLCO with preservation, or at most a mild reduction, in lung volumes, with the exception of SScPAH where disproportionate reduction of DLCO is the rule.
- In PH due to hypoxic lung disease, there may be severe airflow obstruction (FEV$_1$/FVC < 50%), $\downarrow$ (ILD) or $\uparrow$ (emphysema) lung volumes and substantially reduced DLCO, and $\uparrow$ or normal PaCO$_2$.

- In mild to moderate PAH, the PaO_2 is normal or only slightly reduced. $PaCO_2$ may be reduced due to alveolar hyperventilation.
- A low PaO_2 is found in severe lung disease, severe PAH and significant congenital cardiac shunts.
- Reversible airflow obstruction due to coexistent, non-associated asthma or bronchitis may be found in PAH patients and should be treated to try to improve symptoms.

Blood tests

Various blood tests are helpful in characterizing the type of PAH, and serum markers (e.g. NT-proBNP and BNP) are used to help evaluate the impact of PAH on RV function and monitoring RV function and response to therapy.

Routine tests in evaluating patients with PAH include: immunological tests for CTD, LFTs, HIV status, tests for inflammation, renal function, haematological tests, and thyroid function.

NT-proBNP and BNP

These natriuretic peptides are released in response to pressure and volume overload of the ventricles. Falling levels of NT-proBNP correlate with improving haemodynamics and survival while increasing levels correlate with clinical deterioration. There is no widely agreed level of NT-proBNP which is helpful for diagnosing or excluding PAH because the level reflects RV stress rather than mPAP.

Patients should have regular monitoring of NT-proBNP. One aim of treatment is to achieve a decrease and, if possible, normalization of the level.

Troponin

This is released from damaged myocardial cells and is now used to risk stratify and diagnose patients presenting with suspected MI. Raised troponin levels are found in various conditions including acute heart failure and PE. Its role in PAH requires clarification; however, raised levels are associated with a very poor prognosis. With the increasing availability of high sensitivity assays, it is likely that a higher proportion of patients will be found to have evidence of chronic myocardial damage due to pressure overload.

Genetic testing

Associations between mutations of *BMPR2* and *ALK1* and PAH have been identified, however, many mutations have been identified and testing only for known mutations can miss hereditable forms of PAH. In practice, therefore, a 3-generation FH is taken and if premature death from PAH or breathlessness is identified or another case of PAH is found, then genetic testing should be undertaken. If material is available from more than one family member with PAH then the probability of identifying the mutation is ↑ substantially.

V/Q scanning

A normal V/Q scan excludes CTEPH and is extremely useful where present. Many centres will only scan patients with a normal CXR. A mismatch between the inhaled (ventilation, V) radioisotope (krypton-81m) and the injected (perfusion, Q) radioisotope (technetium-labelled, albumin macroaggregates) is suggestive of intraluminal vascular obstruction. V/Q scanning is a relatively low radiation dose examination of 1–2mSV.

- In CTEPH multiple, bilateral segmental mismatched ventilation:perfusion defects (abnormal perfusion with normal ventilation) may be seen (Fig. 30.3).
- When the CXR is normal and the pretest probability of CTEPH is low, a normal V/Q scan has a very high negative predictive value (>91%) and effectively excludes PE and CTEPH.
- A large proportion of patients (70%) may have 'intermediate' or 'low' probability results. 33% and 12% of these respectively may have PEs on pulmonary angiography.
- Matched defects may also occur in PEs if the PE results in infarction, and this reduces the positive predictive value from 88%.
- Compared to CTPA, V:Q scanning has a higher sensitivity, is less expensive, more widely available, and is the recommended screening test to exclude CTEPH. The complete absence of perfusion of one lung may be due to malignancy, mediastinal fibrosis, or vasculitis.
- Defects in perfusion are caused by a variety of lung conditions including infection, bullous emphysema, previous pulmonary infarction, and scarring, but in these cases of parenchymal lung disease, there will be a matched ventilation defect.
- In PAH, the V:Q scan may be normal or show patchy non-segmental defects.
- V:Q scanning is accurate when negative, i.e. in excluding CTEPH.

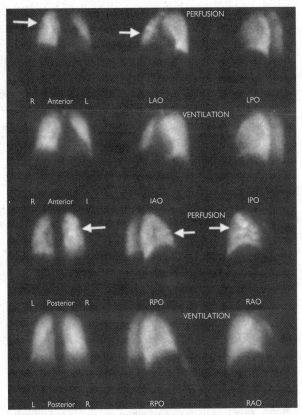

Fig. 30.3 Ventilation perfusion scan of a patient with thromboembolic disease. The 1st series are perfusion images and immediately below these are the corresponding ventilation images. The 3rd and 4th series are further perfusion and ventilation images respectively. Arrows point to some of the defects in the perfusion images for which there are no corresponding defects on the corresponding ventilation images. This technique is highly sensitive and may be positive even when the CTPA is normal.

High resolution computed tomography

HRCT lung scanning in PAH

A normal CTPA does not exclude PAH.

In IPAH the features may include:
- Mural calcific deposits in the proximal PAs in very chronic PAH.
- Mosaic attenuation– which must be differentiated from lung inhomogeneity from parenchymal disease, wedge-shaped perfusion deficits in CTEPH, and centrilobular oedema, lymphadenopathy, ↑ septal lines and pleural effusions in PVOD/PCH.
- Lymphadenopathy is unusual except in sarcoid and CTD, but is common in PVOD.
- Pleural effusions in advanced heart failure or earlier in PVOD.

The scan may also show features consistent with PAH: RV hypertrophy or dilatation, MPA >aorta diameter, pericardial effusion, or other abnormalities complicating the diagnosis—parenchymal lung disease, mediastinal abnormalities, lymphadenopathy, extrinsic compression of the PAs, oesophageal dilatation in SSc, and left heart disease.

HRCT scanning in ILD

HRCT scanning is helpful in assessing the extent of ILD and emphysema and other structural lung disease (Fig. 26.2). A normal HRCT scan excludes significant fibrosis. The signs include:
- Ground-glass opacification.
- Fine reticular pattern superimposed.
- Traction bronchiectasis and architectural distortion.
- Honeycombing of the lungs.
- Enlarged mediastinal lymph nodes.
- Dilated oesophagus in IPF complicating SSc.

Although the ratio of the diameter of the main PA:aortic diameter is typical in PH, PA dilatation in isolation is unreliable and is often abnormal in pulmonary fibrosis.

In IPF (UIP) changes are in the basal, posterior and peripheral areas.

In PVOD and PCH, characterized by obstructions of the pulmonary septal veins and venules, the HRCT appearances include:
- Poorly defined centrilobular ground-glass opacities.
- Smooth thickened interlobular septa.
- Mediastinal lymph nodes.

Pulmonary angiography and magnetic resonance scanning

Multislice (multidetector) CTPA

This has replaced invasive pulmonary angiography in many centres. Surgeons performing PEA in the UK also like imaging of subsegmental PAs using at least 2 imaging modalities (CTPA, invasive pulmonary angiography or MRPA) to visualize small subsegmental PAs.

- In IPAH, the PAs are enlarged (main PA >aorta) and changes may be gross, there are no features of CTEPH—described on 📖 p.148
- Secondary effects of PH seen on CTPA include: dilatation of the RV, reflux of contrast medium down the IVC, pleural and pericardial effusions, and deviation of the IVS to the left.
- Laminated 'thrombus' in the walls of proximal pulmonary vasculature is the hallmark of operable CTEPH (as opposed to intraluminal abnormalities in acute PE)
- Absent vessels—each major vessel should trifurcate, the presence of bronchi with no associated vessel is helpful in identifying missing vessels (Figs. 30.4 and 30.5).
- Webs—important, these occur at branch points, thus impair perfusion to multiple segments.
- Bronchial/systemic arterial collaterals.
- Additional information is available by looking at 'lung windows' which show areas of reduced perfusion (mosaic perfusion pattern) and help to focus attention on absent vessels that may be otherwise missed.
- The scan may in some cases, show other abnormalities accounting for the patient's clinical presentation, e.g. aortic aneurysm, intrathoracic mass.

The pitfalls of CTPA include poor opacification of the pulmonary arterial tree due to obesity or insufficient contrast delivery; breathing and cardiac movement may result in an apparent intraluminal defect. Complications of CTPA include contrast reactions and renal impairment.

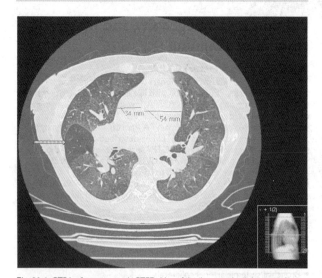

Fig. 30.4 CTPA of a patient with CTED. Use of the 'lung window' shows perfusion, thus mosaic perfusion patterns are evident in this patient—particularly striking at the hatched arrow, where the parenchyma is much blacker and there is a paucity of vessels. Supporting evidence is seen from the enlarged main pulmonary artery.

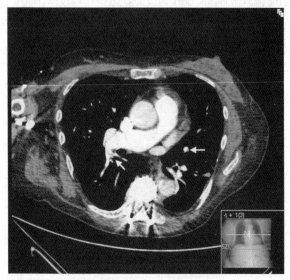

Fig. 30.5 CTPA of a patient with CTED. Irregular filling defects adherent to the internal wall of the arteries rather than centrally placed arrows.

Conventional invasive pulmonary angiography

Invasive pulmonary angiography can be done at the same time as RHC and is the gold standard diagnostic investigation. In specialist centres, performed by experienced operators in patients with normal or near normal renal function and modern contrast media, it is a low-risk procedure (<1:1000 serious risk). Renal function should be checked both before and after the procedure.

Invasive pulmonary angiography provides excellent visualization of the PAs and arterioles in CTEPH when considering suitability for PEA (Fig. 30.6). These include:

- Pouching defect (saccular stop) of the PA.
- Transverse webs or bands tethering the arterial lumen.
- Irregularities of the arterial wall.
- Abrupt change in arterial calibre.
- Absence of lobar arterial branches with parenchymal defects in these territories.

Other conditions, including pulmonary arteriovenous malformations and vasculitis, may be found.

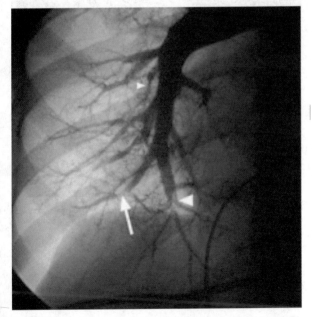

Fig. 30.6 Invasive pulmonary angiogram showing embolic obstruction in the right PA.

MR pulmonary angiography

Contrast-enhanced MRA is used to detect PEs with a sensitivity of 77–100% and specificity of 62–98% depending on the location of the thrombus. The diagnostic accuracy is greater for central thrombi. MRA is used for patients who cannot have a contrast-enhanced CTPA because of renal impairment or contrast allergy. No radiation is involved but its use in pregnancy is controversial.

The precise role of MRA in CTEPH is being established; it is presently accepted as a supporting investigation where other studies have suggested the presence of CTEPH, and provides additional information in respect of operability (Fig. 30.7).

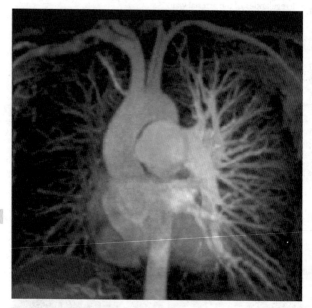

Fig. 30.7 Figure showing that in addition to cardiac information, the pulmonary vascular tree can be imaged, offering the potential to simplify the diagnostic routine.

Cardiac magnetic resonance imaging (CMR)

MRI provides high-quality images of the RV and PAs and information on blood flow and estimates of PAP, but is not sufficiently accurate for diagnosis or screening for PAH.

CMR is useful to assess haemodynamics and anatomy in CHD in both the heart and great vessels.

CMR is used to assess both LV and RV systolic and diastolic function and ventricular mass, and pericardial disease.

The advantages of CMR include: rapid scanning sequences, useful haemodynamic and anatomical information, safety because there is no ionizing radiation, and good spatial resolution (Figs. 30.8 and 30.9).

The disadvantages include the claustrophobic scanner which some patients cannot tolerate, the difficulty in monitoring sick patients, their expense, and patients with some metallic prostheses cannot be scanned. These include most pacemakers (MRI safe pacemakers are now available) and implantable cardioverter defibrillators and LV assist devices.

The detail of the cardiac anatomy available on CMR scanning means that this technique is essential in patients with complex CHD.

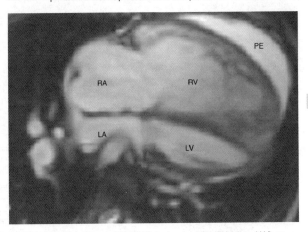

Fig. 30.8 CMR of the heart in PAH. All four chambers (RA, RV, LA, and LV) can be seen in any orientation. Here the left heart is obviously compressed by the enlarged right heart, a prognostically significant pericardial effusion (PE) is evident. The greater detail of the RV free wall when compared to echo may help improve understanding of the cardiac response to pulmonary hypertension.

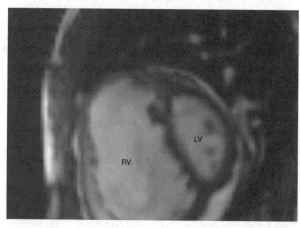

Fig. 30.9 CMR of the heart in PAH. This figure shows a short-axis cut through the RV and LV, again showing how the LV is compressed by the enlarged RV. Similar slices can be obtained from base to apex and the information from each summated to describe the function of the heart throughout systole and diastole.

Echocardiography

TTE provides useful information on various structural heart diseases which can cause PH: LV and RV structure, dimensions and function, valve abnormalities, and a significant ASD or VSD can be evaluated.

Doppler echocardiography

RV systolic pressure (TRV)

This is the most useful non-invasive method for screening for PAH but has significant limitations.

RVSP is calculated from the TRV. TRV (m/s) is derived from continuous wave Doppler ultrasound mapping of the tricuspid regurgitant jet. TRV reflects RV:RA pressure difference. If there is no pulmonary stenosis, RVSP is equal to PASP:

From Bernoulli we know PASP = RVSP = $4(TRV)^2$ + RAP

In patients with a normal jugular venous pressure (JVP), an RAP value of 5cm is used.

Inaccuracies in estimated PASP are due to:
- Technical and operator problems.
- Assumption of the RAP from the JVP or IVC reactivity.
- Magnification of an initial inaccuracy in the Doppler velocity measurement which is squared and multiplied by 4 in the Bernoulli equation.
- Severe 'free-flow' TR which invalidates the Bernoulli equation. TVR will underestimate the transtricuspid pressure.

When used to screen for PAH and compared to cardiac catheterization, Doppler echocardiography has a substantial false positive rate (overestimating PASP by >20% in 50% of patients) and false negative (underestimating PASP by >10mmHg) in 50% of patients.

PASP may be higher (>40mmHg) in obese and elderly patients without PAH. Another drawback of using TVR is that it estimates PASP rather than mPAP which is used for diagnosis and management of PAH.

Because of the constant relationship between PASP and mPAP, mPAP can be calculated from 0.61 × PASP + 2mmHg.

TRV: Doppler estimates of TR velocity (m/sec) are load dependent and therefore depend on the fluid status of the patient.

The upper limit of normal for PASP = 36 mmHg (TRV = 2.8m/s).

Echocardiography and screening for PAH

Echocardiography is inaccurate for screening for mild, asymptomatic PAH.

The accuracy of echocardiography depends on the population under study, and technical and operator factors (Table 30.1):
- The higher the TVR, the more likely that the patient will have PH (a lower false positive rate and a higher diagnostic accuracy).
- As with other screening tests, there is a trade-off between sensitivity and specificity.
- There is a high false positive rate (45%) if cut-off values of TVR >2.5m/s in symptomatic patients or <3.2m/s, with or without symptoms, are used.
- Mild PAH is commonly associated with a TVR of 2.8–3.4m/s, the grey area where test reliability is worst.
- Very high or very low values of TVR are usually reliable.
- Inability to document TRV due to absence of regurgitation does not exclude PH.

There is a poor correlation between echocardiographic estimates of PASP and symptoms, exercise response, or prognosis. This is because TVR does not accurately reflect RV function which is the major determinant of functional class and prognosis. (Figs. 30.10, 30.11, and 30.19).

Table 30.1 Arbitrary criteria of estimating the presence of PH based on TVR and estimated PASP from echocardiography using a normal RAP = 5mmHg

TVR (m/s)	PASP (mmHg)	Other findings	PH probability
≤2.8	≤36	Nil	Very low
≤2.8	≤36	Yes	Medium
2.9–3.3	37–50	Yes/no	Medium
>3.4	50	Yes/no	High

Other echocardiographic derived variables have been used to diagnose PH. Those assessing the effects of PH on the RV include RV function and size, abnormal shape and function of the IVS, ↑ RV wall thickness; these are useful but reflect RV damage and therefore are not suitable for screening.

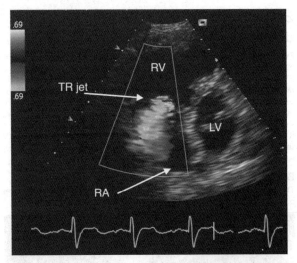

Fig. 30.10 (Also see Colour plate 2.) Short axis echocardiographic view at the level of the tricuspid valve with colour flow Doppler showing tricuspid valve regurgitation during systole. This can be used to estimate the optimal angle for determining the tricuspid gradient. LV = left ventricle. RV = right ventricle.

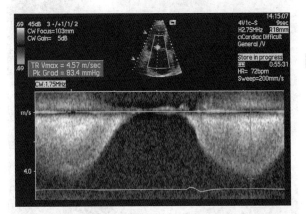

Fig. 30.11 (Also see Colour plate 3.) Estimating pulmonary pressure using echocardiography. Doppler signals are used to determine the velocity with which blood regurgitates through the tricuspid valve during systole. 70% of normal people have enough regurgitation to use this technique, the frequency is higher in PAH. Doppler relies on the change in frequency of reflected sound waves proportional to the velocity of the target. The Bernoulli equation ($P = 4V^2$ where P = pressure and V = velocity) describes this relationship. Thus the difference between right ventricular systolic pressure and right atrial systolic pressure can be directly measured. The technique is quite error prone, with a standard deviation of ±20mmHg.

Echocardiographic assessment of the RV

Estimating the size of the RV is inaccurate because of its complex shape. Normally, the anterior RV wall is thin (3–5mm) and the diameter of the RV is <1/3 of the LV. Most echo labs estimate the size of the RV qualitatively as normal; or slightly, moderately (the same size as the LV) or severely (bigger than the LV) enlarged. Actual measurements are more useful—the RV internal diameter at 0.5–1cm below the tricuspid valve should be compared to the LV internal diameter below the mitral valve. RV function is also graded qualitatively. This subjective assessment of RV size and function means that serial assessments by different observers may be unreliable.

Pericardial effusion

The presence and size of a pericardial effusion is a poor prognostic sign occurring in severe RV failure (see Figs. 30.12 and 30.13).

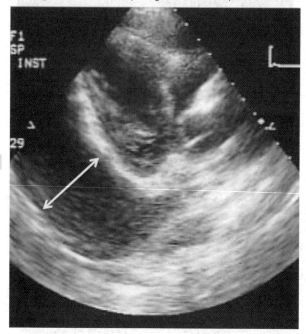

Fig. 30.12 Echocardiogram showing a pericardial effusion (PE). These are readily identifiable when present in PAH patients and indicate that the right ventricle has failed. They are invariably transudates and do not cause tamponade. Note the very large RV and RV with bowing of the septum into the LV (arrow).

Geometric measurements of RV function

These all share similar inherent limitations because volumetric approximations of the RV are load dependent and measurements are complicated by RV geometry. These include RV area, fractional area change (from the 4-chamber view), RV diameters (RVA1 just below the tricuspid valve, RVD2 the transverse diameter 1/3 of the way into the ventricle, RVD3 the longitudinal distance apex to tricuspid valve), and outflow tract diameters.

The normal values for some measures depend on how they are performed, thus the basal diameter of the RV is up to 2.8cm in the 4-chamber view, and up to 5.4cm in the parasternal long-axis view of the RV inflow tract (Figs. 30.13 and 30.14).

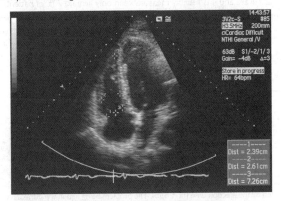

Fig. 30.13 Figure showing substantial pericardial effusion (arrow).

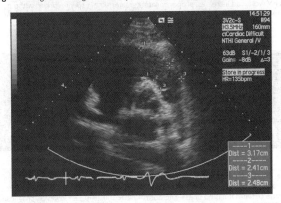

Fig. 30.14 Echocardiographic assessment of the right ventricular outflow tract (RVOT). The short-axis view of the aortic valve is used as an anatomical marker with the pulmonary valve in view. Diameter 1 is taken from the commissure of the NC cusp to the wall of the RVOT in line with the commissure, Diameter 3 underneath the pulmonary valve and diameter 2 the shortest distance half way between the two on the minor axis. Clearly demonstrating how limited our echocardiographic representation of the complexity of the RV is.

Load 'independent' measures of RV performance

Myocardial performance index (MPI; Tei index)

This is a combination of systolic and diastolic measurements. The measure relies on the fact that an efficient ventricle wastes relatively little time on non-ejecting contraction and relaxation. (Figs. 30.15 and 30.16).

- Thus Tei = isovolumic contraction plus relaxation time (ms) divided by ejection time (ms), normal 0.28–0.32.
- Values >0.88 predict poor prognosis.
- It is reproducible and quick to calculate but has limitations, in particular calculating isovolumic times, which are very short in the normal RV, is inaccurate and it is reliably measurable in only around 70% of patients.

Contraction time – flow time = isovolumic contraction + relaxation time

Thus (a – b)/b = Tei index or MPI

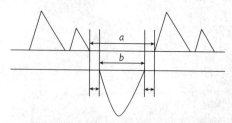

Fig. 30.15 Line drawing showing the concept behind the TEI index. The proportion of RV active systole taken up with isovolumetric contraction and relaxation is divided by the ejection time [(a – b)/b]. The problem being that in the normal RV it may be almost impossible to see any evidence of isovolumetric activity. In theory, as RV workload increases, proportionately greater time is spent working without forward flow. This is used as a measure of volume independent RV function and correlates with RVEF as measured on CMR.

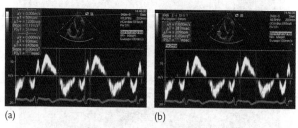

(a)   (b)

Fig. 30.16 Tissue Doppler measurement of isovolumic contraction and relaxation (a) and ejection time (b)—these timings are used to calculate the TEI index. Note as a ratio of times it has no units—the normal range is 0.28–0.32. However, prognosis in PAH is not known to be adversely affected below 0.88.

Tricuspid annular plane systolic excursion (TAPSE)

TAPSE is a distance measure, of the excursion of the lateral tricuspid annulus toward the apex during systole, it is highly angle dependent. TAPSE is a simple and easily obtained measurement and correlates with radionuclide ventriculographic measurements of radionuclide ejection fraction and MRI-derived volumes (Fig. 30.17).

- TAPSE is measured in the apical 4-chamber view.
- The normal TAPSE value is >16mm, commonly in well functioning RVs it exceeds 20mm.
- TAPSE falls as RV function is impaired, but may paradoxically increase as tricuspid regurgitation becomes more severe.
- TAPSE only reflects longitudinal function, so it does not always accurately reflect RV function.
- Measurement may be inaccurate if the 4-chamber view is off axis, or radial contraction of the RV moves the tricuspid annulus out of the M-mode line.

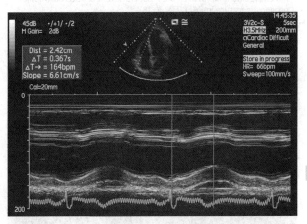

Fig. 30.17 TAPSE is another volume independent measure of RV function. Longitudinal contraction dominates in the RV thus the movement of the tricuspid annulus toward the apex in cm varies as RV function varies. Unlike TEI this measure is highly angle dependent but has the advantage of being readily measurable in all patients. The lower limit of normal is 1.5cm; however, prognosis in PAH is adversely affected once TAPSE falls below 2.0cm, making this a more sensitive measure than TEI.

Tricuspid annulus velocity

The velocity of movement of the myocardium close to the TV can be assessed using angle dependent (tissue Doppler) and non-angle dependent (speckled tracking) methods.

- In well functioning RVs the velocity of systolic movement is well preserved (>11.5cm/s)—this is reported as the S wave velocity.
- S-wave velocity correlates with radionuclide ventriculography measurements of RV ejection fraction.
- A systolic annular velocity of <11.5cm/s has a sensitivity of 90% and a specificity of 85% for predicting RV ejection fraction <45%.

RV diastolic function

RV diastolic function can be assessed by Doppler interrogation of tricuspid, hepatic, and superior vena cava inflow patterns.

- As in LV diastolic dysfunction one of the most reliable findings is atrial enlargement—normal $13.5\pm2cm^2$
- RA enlargement has proven the most consistent echocardiographic prognostic feature in PAH (Fig. 30.18).

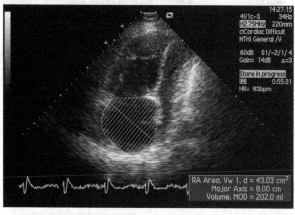

Fig. 30.18 Assessment of right atrial area in the 4-chamber view at the onset of systole. The precise normal value is being reviewed—18cm² has been accepted on the basis of small studies, however, it is recognized that this is a little generous and fails to account for variable body size; 9cm²/m² is probably more accurate. RA enlargement occurs early in the development of pulmonary hypertension and thus should be assessed in all patients undergoing echocardiography.

Features of PH on the RV include:

- Dilatation of the RV. The moderator band will be seen traversing the RV and this may complicate measurements of the IVS.
- Increases in basal diameter of the RV and dilatation of the tricuspid annulus.
- Flattening and displacement of the IVS.
- Increased TRV >3.2cm/s (values of 2.8–3.2cm/s have a lower predictive accuracy).
- Dilatation of the RV outflow tract, main PA, RA area.
- Pericardial effusion which is a poor prognostic sign in PH.

3D echocardiography may provide more consistent and repeatable information.

Normal RV measurements (Table 30.2)

Table 30.2 Normal measurements for RV variables

Variable	Normal
TRV (m/s)	<2.6
RAP (mmHg)	<5
RV MPI Tei index	<0.28–0.32
TAPSE (mm)	>16

RAP, right atrial pressure; RV MPI Tei index, right ventricular myocardial performance index; TAPSE, tricuspid annular plane systolic excursion; TRV, tricuspid valve regurgitant jet velocity.

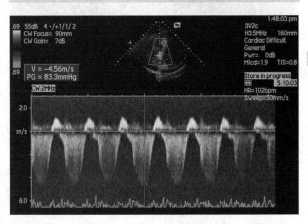

Fig. 30.19 (Also see Colour plate 4.) Tricuspid velocity assessment using Doppler. Note unless a clear envelope of regurgitant signal is available, estimates of the maximum velocity can be very inaccurate. The sweep speed should be at least 50mm/s and use of colour rather than greyscale improves the ability to see the signal. The estimate is highly angle dependent and underestimation occurs if alignment is incorrect. Overestimation may occur if the probe is causing discomfort or the patient is holding their breath in expiration causing a 'Valsalva' type phenomenon.

Echocardiography to assess PH due to left heart disease

Echocardiography is very helpful in the assessment of PH due to left heart disease. It aids diagnosis of:

- LV systolic and/or diastolic dysfunction.
- LV and LA dimensions.
- Valvar heart disease.
- Pericardial disease.
- CHD, including ASD, PFO, and VSD.

The impact of RV enlargement on the LV should not be overlooked when assessing RV function. Pressure-loaded RVs compress the LV. This can be assessed either by considering the shape of the LV in the short-axis view (Eccentricity index) or considering the relative diameters of the RV (RVA1 in the 4-chamber view) and the LV—measured from the parasternal long-axis view—the RV diameter should be less than the LV diameter in normal patients.

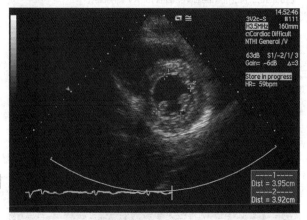

Fig. 30.20 Eccentricity index measurement. From the short-axis view at the level of the papillary muscles the LV should appear as a near perfect circle. The minor axis (1) should be equal to the major axis (2) thus D2/D1 should equal unity in both systole and diastole. Normal findings are shown here, but as seen in Fig. 14.4 where septal flattening has occurred D2 significantly exceeds D1.

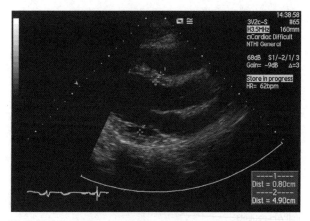

Fig. 30.21 LV internal diameter assessed in the parasternal long-axis view. In normal people RVA1 <LVID, as PH progresses enlargement of the RV is evident and in response to treatment the RV may shrink. The changing relationship between RVA1 and LVID can be used to monitor such changes over time.

3D echocardiography

The role of 3D echocardiography is unclear. With advances, we can expect that 3D echocardiography will provide reliable estimates of the RV volume in systole and diastole, and as frame rate increases we should be able to analyse strain (magnitude of local contraction) in all regions of the right ventricle simultaneously. We should also be able to assess RA volumes (likely to correlate better with prognosis than RA area) and volume of tricuspid regurgitation.

Stress echocardiography

Exercise stress echocardiography should provide more accurate information on RV functional reserve compared to a resting study. The role of exercise echocardiography in diagnosis and management of PAH is, however, unclear because there is no universally accepted validated definition of normal or abnormal values, the derived measurement is PASP rather than mPAP which is used for diagnosis of PAH, and there are a number of confounding factors influencing the derived PASP: lack of reproducibility of results, age, gender, weight, physical fitness, ability to exercise due to associated musculoskeletal impairment, delay in obtaining peak exercise images from either treadmill or cycle, drug effects, which complicate interpretation of the result.

An arbitrarily defined value for a normal exercise maximum PASP of 40mmHg has been defined but this has not been widely adopted. Further data evaluating the prognostic value of exercise Doppler echocardiography are required.

The majority of patients with PAH are echogenic and the data necessary for diagnosis are usually available from TTE.

TOE is rarely necessary for a diagnosis of PAH, but can be useful where shunts require definition.

Non-invasive exercise testing

Cardiopulmonary exercise testing (CPET)

CPET measures integrated cardiopulmonary performance at rest and during exercise. The role of CPET for diagnosis is unclear.

In PAH there is impairment of gas exchange due to abnormal ventilation-perfusion, and CO limitation during exercise. Exercise capacity is reduced and peak O_2 uptake (VO_{2peak}) is around 40% of normal in most patients with PAH. There may also be a reduced lactic acidosis threshold, high LAT/VO_{2peak} ratio (opposite to deconditioning), ↓ mixed venous O_2 at maximum exercise, ↑ ventilatory equivalents for O_2 and CO_2 (VE/VCO_2 slope).

CPET may be used to monitor the response to treatment and several CPET variables correlate with survival (ventilatory equivalents for O_2 and CO_2 correlate with disease severity).

The peak systolic BP and VO_{2max} are independent predictors of survival in IPAH patients.

6MWD correlates with CPET and is much easier to perform and interpret and is therefore used both clinically and as an endpoint in drug trials.

The method is currently not widely used to aid diagnosis or monitoring prognosis or response to treatment because of interobserver variability and lack of standardization between CPET laboratories. However, at the extremes useful information is available; hence the European Society of Cardiology (ESC) and the European Respiratory Society (ERS) guidelines do include CPET as one of the potential methods of assessing adequacy of response to therapy.

6MWD

This is commonly used as a trial endpoint but there are inherent limitations. There is only an approximate correlation of the 6MWD with VO_{2max} and body mass and age should be incorporated into the calculation. 6MWD is a test of fitness, musculoskeletal fitness, and flexibility.

The 6MWD has to be interpreted with caution in older less fit patients who may have arthritic problems, and CTD-PAH where there may be leg and foot ulceration and muscular pain.

6WMD is mainly a measure of aerobic performance. As with most forms of exercise testing, 6MWD improves with training and familiarity with the test.

Most importantly, change in 6MWD in response to therapy has never been shown to predict prognosis. 6MWD can therefore be thought of as analogous to an assessment of well-being—those who are well are more likely to survive, minor changes in degree of wellness do not predict survival. However, modest changes in 6MWD (40m) correlate with quality of life changes.

Exercise tests for ischaemic heart disease

The recent NICE guidance has highlighted the inaccuracy of standard exercise testing for the exclusion of IHD, thus for the purposes of excluding IHD in patients with PH standard guidance would apply—electron beam CT with or without CT coronary angiography for low-risk patients. Myocardial perfusion imaging or stress echocardiography for moderate risk patients, and invasive angiography for those with a significant (>60%) pre-test probability.

Further reading

National Institute for Health and Clinical Excellence Guideline CG126. *Management of stable angina*. Issue date July 2011. London: National Institute for Health and Clinical Excellence.

ESC Guidelines on the management of stable angina sectors: Executive summary. *Eur Heart J* 2006; **27**:1341–1381.

Cardiac catheterization

Coronary angiography

This is indicated in patients:
- With angina refractory to medical treatment.
- Aged >50 with an intermediate probability of coronary heart disease.
- With CTEPH who are considered for PEA.
- Being assessed for double LT.

The risks of coronary angiography are similar in PAH patients as in non-PAH patients.

Cardiac catheterization

RHC is essential for diagnosis of PH.

Left heart disease is common in some types of PAH.

Left heart catheterization may also be necessary to obtain the LVEDP if the PCWP is unreliable, and to investigate the possibility of restriction or constriction. Coronary angiography may be necessary to exclude left heart pathology and coronary heart disease causing post-capillary PH.

Right heart catheterization

RHC is essential to:
- Confirm or exclude PH.
- To characterize it and distinguish it from post-capillary PH where the PCWP is ≥16mm Hg.
- Test for vasoreactivity.
- Invasive pulmonary angiography can be done at the same time.

RHC is performed from the neck, antecubital fossa, or groin, using a Swan–Ganz thermodilution catheter, which allows calculation of both thermodilution CO and Fick CO. The catheter has 4 ports:
- Balloon tip.
- Proximal port.
- Distal port which sits in the PA.
- Thermistor at the distal end of the catheter.

The advantage of using the groin, preferred by most cardiologists, is that coronary angiography, left heart catheterization to measure the LVEDP in cases of questionable accuracy of the PCWP, pulmonary angiography, and coronary intervention, can be done conveniently at the same time. The procedure may be technically more difficult in patients who cannot lie flat because of breathlessness, in patients with diffuse scleroderma (local skin thickening) and in others with severe associated medical conditions. Alternately the radial can be used in association with the antecubital fossa, though radial cannulation is relatively contraindicated in systemic sclerosis because of the higher rate of forearm ischaemia associated with radial artery trauma in these patients.

Complications of RHC using balloon catheters

Serious complications

The combined risk of MI, stroke, death, pulmonary haemorrhage, PA rupture, pulmonary infarction, valvular trauma (most commonly tricuspid valve), is 0.1% in experienced centres. Infection and endocarditis are very rare.

Minor complications

Transient arrhythmias during catheter movement in the RA, near the TV and in the RV. Atrial arrhythmias are common if a catheter distends the RA. Persistent AF or ventricular arrhythmias may cause important haemodynamic deterioration in PH but can be avoided with careful technique. Bruising and haematoma formation are uncommon after RHC.

Normal RHC values (Table 30.3)

Table 30.3 Normal measurements for RHC variables

Variable	Value
mRAP	0–5 mmHg
RVEDP	<5mmHg
PASP	20±4/8±3mmHg
mPAP	14±3mmHg
PCWP	≤15mmHg
mixed venous O_2 saturation	65–70%
CO	4–6L/min
CI (CO/BSA)	2.5–3.5L/min/m^2
PVR	240 dynes.sec.cm^{-5}

BSA, body surface area; CI, cardiac index; CO, cardiac output; mPAP, mean pulmonary artery pressure; mRAP, mean right atrial pressure; PAP, pulmonary artery pressure; PCWP, mean pulmonary artery capillary wedge pressure; PVR, pulmonary vascular resistance; RVEDP, right ventricular end-diastolic pressure.

Technique of Swan–Ganz catheterization

- The procedure is best performed with radiography, though from the neck this is not mandatory.
- The patient must be comfortable and relaxed to avoid spurious increases in mPAP, systemic BP, HR, and CO.
- If the patient cannot lie flat comfortably, extra pillows are required.
- Patients who require continuous O_2 should have an O_2 mask with their usual O_2 flow rate.
- The zero (balance) is achieved by placing the patient end of the manometer at the patient's mid thorax (mid RA). Previous studies have also used 10cm above the bed, or 5cm below the sternum.

- It is important to check and recheck the zero if the recordings do not make sense or appear unexpectedly high or low compared to clinical assessment, echocardiographic estimations of PAP, or previous catheter findings. The catheter should be well flushed, and the balloon tested and deflated prior to insertion. The balloon is inflated after the catheter tip has passed through the sheath to avoid the catheter tip getting trapped in small vein side branches and an inflated balloon reduces the risk of vascular trauma.
- Record pressures in RA, RV, main PA, and wedge.
- A high mRAP ≥10mmHg, reflects severe RV impairment. Also consider pericardial constriction.
- mRAP <0mmHg reflects dehydration but check 'zero'.
- RVEDP ≥10mmHg may reflect RV failure, constriction or restriction.
- mPAP ≥25mmHg is diagnostic of PH, but does not indicate the cause.
- To obtain the PCWP, advance the balloon inflated tip gently and slowly in the wedge position while screening. If no suitable wedge recording is obtained, deflate and then gradually inflate the balloon to see if it 'catches' in a suitable vessel. If no suitable PCWP is obtained try a different position or try the other lung.
- PCWP >15mmHg reflects a high LVEDP and/or LA pressure due to LV myocardial impairment due to ischaemia and/or infarction, systemic hypertension, myocardial disease due to any cause, valvular disease, constriction (Fig. 30.24), restriction, amyloid.
- If there is any doubt about the accuracy or reliability of the PCPW (difficulty in finding a suitable position, large respiratory swings in patients with lung disease), the LV should be catheterized to obtain the LVEDP (Fig. 30.23).
- Mitral stenosis will cause a high PCWP but a normal LVEDP (Fig. 30.23).
- Supplemental O_2 should be given to hypoxaemic patients with high mPAP to see if the mPAP falls with O_2.
- A high PA O_2 saturation >80%, particularly with a mPAP >25mmHg and a high CO, might reflect left-to-right intracardiac and extracardiac arteriovenous shunts, high output states (thyrotoxicosis). These should be investigated with a full saturation run and further imaging; in any event a SVC saturation should be obtained to exclude shunts in patients with PH.
- A low PA O_2 saturation <60% may reflect ↑ tissue oxygen extraction but more commonly a low CO.
- Thermodilution CO is done by injecting 10mL of ice cold saline into the proximal port of the Swan–Ganz catheter. The rate of temperature change detected by the thermistor at the catheter tip reflects the cardiac output. A CO computer produces the CO measurement.
- The thermodilution CO is the average of 3 consecutive samples within 10% of each other. Sources of error include: moderate and severe TR which allows some of the bolus to leak back into the RA; septal defects, insufficient temperature difference between injectate and PA blood temperature. An important source of error, if the right internal jugular approach is used, is if the proximal port is within the delivery sheath, since the injectate does not arrive in the RA as a single bolus. The presence of shunts may render Fick a more appropriate way of measuring CO. Thermodilution is inaccurate at the extremes of CO (<3L/min or >9L/min).

Fick principle

The Fick principle uses the difference in O_2 content in the arterial and venous system to measure flow. In the absence of an intracardiac shunt, the saturations in the PA and a systemic artery are used to determine the systemic CO. Each gram of Hb carries 1.34mL of O_2.

One of the very important advantages of the Fick approach to measuring CO is the ability to measure relative flows, where shunts are present. The mixed venous saturation can also be assessed as:

$$(3 \times SVC \text{ sat} + IVC \text{ sat})/4$$

This allows systemic flow—from aorta vs mixed venous saturations, pulmonary flow from pulmonary venous vs pulmonary arterial saturations, and right-to-left shunts—pulmonary venous vs aortic saturations, to be measured.

Oxygen content of the blood = oxygen saturation x haemoglobin $\times$ 1.34

O_2 consumption is derived from body mass and HR.

An assumed value for VO_2 of 125mL O_2/min/m^2 body surface area is often used, but for accuracy O_2 consumption should be measured directly.

The Fick formula is:

$$CO = \frac{O_2 \text{ consumption (mL/min)}}{[A - VO_2] \times 1.34mL/g \times Hgb(9g/dL) \times 10(dL/L)}$$

where $A - VO_2$ is the difference in O_2 saturation between the arterial and venous circulation.

Data recorded at RHC and technique

- HR, BP, height and weight (to calculate BSA and CI), systemic BP, Hb, arterial (oximeter or direct arterial sample) and mixed venous (PA) oxygen saturation, mRAP, RVP, PAP (systolic, diastolic, and mPAP), PCWP, and PVR (mPAP − PCWP/CO).
- The catheter must be in the PA when aspirating blood for the PA sample.
- All recordings should be made at end-expiration (closest to zero net intrathoracic pressure) (Fig. 30.22).
- The CO measured by both Fick and in triplicate by thermodilution averaging 3 consecutive recordings within 10% of each other to calculate PVR.
- O_2 should be given to patients with an arterial saturation <92% to increase the arterial O_2 saturation to >95% to see if there is a fall in mPAP.
- It is essential that an accurate zero is obtained because of the major implications of recording a PCWP/LVEDP ≥16mmHg. There may be 'drift of the zero'. Patients with mPCWP/LVEDP >15mmHg would not be diagnosed as PAH and not be treated and their prognosis may be different.

- A full saturation run: oxygen saturation in the IVC, SVC, high, mid, and low RA, RV outflow tract, left and right PA, aortic and if available LA and pulmonary vein should be performed if there is a suspicion of a shunt.

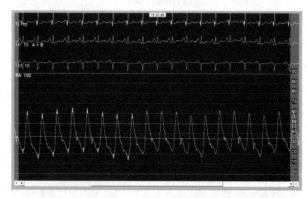

Fig. 30.22 Tracing of pulmonary artery pressure in a patient with PH. At end expiration the PA pressure is 62/23 mean 36mmHg. This does not tell us which of the 5 WHO groups of PH this patient has.

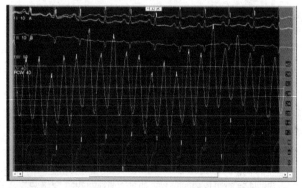

Fig. 30.23 Simultaneous tracing of LVEDP and CW in the same patient as in Fig. 30.22, note the LVEDP is normal (12mmHg) and if only this was assessed one might conclude that the patient had pre-capillary PH. The wedge pressure with an end-expiration value of 32mmHg however shows that this patient has post-capillary PH. In this case due to mitral stenosis (unusually the echocardiogram had not reported this abnormality, though repeat echo after diagnosis was confirmatory).

Prognostic data from RHC

RV function is the main prognostic determinant; grossly abnormal results indicate a poor prognosis, and independent markers of prognosis include:

- CI <2.1L/min/m^2.
- RAP >10mmHg.
- Mixed venous saturation <60%, reflecting low CO and ↑ oxygen extraction.

Conditions to exclude during RHC

Shunting

ASD or other systemic-to-pulmonary shunts are likely if the PA saturation is >80%. In all diagnostic catheters, at the minimum one should demonstrate that SVC saturations are similar to PA saturation. Shunting can occur at various arteriovenous sites and malformations.

Constriction and restriction (Table 30.4)

If RVEDP is high consider restriction or constriction:

- Restriction and constriction are typically associated with a sharp dip and plateau appearance in the LV and RV pressure waveform in early and mid-diastole. This should be recorded at LVEDP range (50mmHg) at fast paper and recording speed.
- Simultaneous LVEDP and RVEDP recorded at 50mm/s, and RV and LV systolic pressure recordings will help distinguish restriction from constriction, and from biventricular failure.
- Findings favouring constriction:
  - The LVEDP-RVEDP is separated by <5mmHg throughout respiratory cycle.
  - The RVEDP is generally >1/3 of the RVSP.
  - The RVSP is usually <55mmHg.
  - In addition there is dissociation of intrathoracic and intracardiac pressure, so LVEDP − PCWP may be >5mmHg in inspiration.
  - There is ventricular interdependence, thus the LV systolic pressure falls in inspiration while the RV systolic pressure rises, with reversal of this pattern in expiration.

Note these final two findings can only be reliably identified with high-fidelity catheters.

In practice therefore one does not rely on any individual technique or test to distinguish restriction from constriction. Important considerations include the filling status of the patient (gross fluid overload may mask respiratory variation in flows in constriction) and massive variations in intrathoracic pressures (e.g. COPD), creating significant variations in flow and intracardiac pressures with respiration.

Table 30.4 Differences between constriction and restriction

	Constriction	Restriction
CXR	Pericardial calcification	None
2D Echo	Small ventricles	Small ventricles
	Normal atria	Dilated atria
	Thick pericardium	Normal pericardium
Doppler	25% fall in mitral 'E' wave on inspiration	Minimal respiratory expiration ↑ MV flow
	PV flow varies >25% with respiration	PV flow does not vary with respiration
Haemodynamics	↑LVEDP = RVEDP	↑LVEDP ≠ RVEDP
	PASP <55mmHg	PASP >55mmHg
	RVEDP/RVSP>1/3	RVEDP/RVSP<1/3
	LVP area ↓ RVP area ↑	Concordant changes only
CT/MRI	Thick pericardium	Normal pericardium
	Septal shift toward LV with inspiration	
Myocardial biopsy	Normal	Abnormal

≠ not equal: in restriction the early and late diastolic pressures in RV and LV are not equal and separate during inspiration during the respiratory cycle because the disease is patchy affecting each ventricle to a different extent. This is in contrast to constriction where LVEDP = RVEDP throughout the cardiac cycle in both inspiration and expiration.

MV, mitral valve.

Lung disease and PH

Mild PH (mPAP <35mmHg), is frequent in advanced lung disease. Patients with 'out of proportion' PH, (breathlessness insufficiently explained by the underlying lung condition alone, and with a mPAP >35mmHg at rest), should be referred to a specialist PH centre.

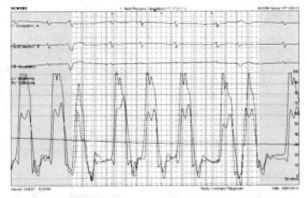

Fig. 30.24 Figure showing RV and LV tracings in a patient with constriction. The RVEDP is 1/3 of the RVSP; the RVSP is a little higher than typical; there is, however, no separation of diastolic pressures; there is a typical dip–plateau diastolic pattern; and there is an increase in RVSP with inspiration with a very minor reduction in LVSP.

Acute vasodilator testing

- Vasodilator testing (VT) should be done at the time of the first diagnostic RHC to identify long-term responders to CCBs.
- Acute vasoreactivity is most likely in anorexigen associated PAH patients (13% are vasoreactive) and IPAH, but is very rare (1%) in other forms of PAH.
- A long-term response to CCB (marked haemodynamic improvement at 3–4 months and New York Heart Association functional class I or II after 1 year) was reported in 6% of PAH-anorexigen patients but was rare in HIV, POPH, CTD (1.6%, 0.7%, and 0.6%, respectively) and absent in PVOD/PCH.
- The prognosis of long-term responders was favourable and related to the underlying cause of PAH.
- Vasoreactive IPAH patients have up to a 95% 5-year survival when treated with CCBs.
- A positive vasodilator response is defined as: a decrease in mPAP of ≥10mmHg to reach an absolute value of <40mmHg with no change or an increase in CO. These criteria are considered the best predictors of long-term response to high-dose oral CCBs (e.g. diltiazem 480mg/d, nifedipine 90mg/d, or amlodipine 20mg/d).
- A long-term vasodilator response is defined as a marked haemodynamic improvement after 3–4 months of CCB therapy (necessitating repeat RHC) and in WHO functional class I or II, at least 1 year after starting CCB. It is not clear which patients respond. Oral CCBs are not always effective in some PAH patients decreasing CO and SVR.
- Though only a small percentage have a persistent response on chronic therapy these fortunate patients have a near normal survival and virtually normal quality of life and exercise tolerance on simple therapy, justifying acute VT.

Recommendations for VT

- Acute VT is recommended in IPAH and anorexigens-associated PAH and POPH and HIV-PAH.
- VT may be considered in CTD-PAH, and CHD-PAH. These patients should be followed-up carefully because they are very unlikely to have a *long-term* response to CCBs and are likely to deteriorate.
- VT response does not predict response to disease-specific treatments.
- Vasoreactivity testing is not recommended in post-capillary PH, PH due to lung diseases, CTEPH, or PH with unclear or multifactorial mechanisms.

Risks of vasodilator testing

CCBs are not recommended for acute VT because of the dangerous falls in CO, SVR, and hypotension, particularly in non-responders.

Therefore, reliable and safe short-acting vasodilators (inhaled NO or inhaled iloprost or IV epoprostenol) are used to test reactivity of vasoconstricted small PAs, a component of the pathophysiology in PAH.

Management of PAH

31 General approach to the management of PAH   **197**

32 Specific therapies for PAH   **209**

General approach to the management of PAH

Introduction 198
Supportive measures 202
Contraception in PAH 203
Risks of pregnancy and contraception 204
Lifestyle issues 206
Elective surgery in patients with PAH 207
Management of arrhythmias 208

Introduction

Aims of treatment

PAH is incurable. The aims of treatment are to:
- Improve symptoms, quality of life, haemodynamics, and heart failure.
- Ideally reverse, or slow down, or at least, stabilize the condition in its early phase.

This necessitates a detailed and comprehensive characterization of the patient's condition and all other associated conditions.

Holistic management and support

This is very important and complex, requiring the skills of various specialists and disciplines, because PAH impacts on various organ systems and the patient's personal, social, and family situations. Patients will find it easier to cope with their condition with wide support, encouragement, and education. There has to be a holistic approach to the patient and their family.

Educating patients about their condition and discussing what may lie around the corner can be done constructively and in a reassuring and non-alarming manner.

Managing patient expectations, hopes, and fears

As with other serious conditions, some patients may want to know all the possible implications of the disease and its management. For patients with advanced and rapidly progressive PAH, this may include medical and surgical treatments including transplantation and palliative care. Others with less severe PAH, may not need or want to know what may lie around the corner, at least during the initial consultations. Although the prognosis for PAH is generally poor and considerably worse when patients progress into WHO class III or, even more seriously, into WHO class IV, the timing of deterioration is difficult to predict. Even if it is not possible to reassure patients, encouragement, practical help and advice, and a positive approach is usually preferred by patients and their family, rather than providing them with gloomy, depressing, unhelpful predictions. The art of the consultation is for the clinician to listen and observe the patient very carefully and sensitively and tailor the tone of the consultation and advice provided to the patient and their mood.

Multidisciplinary multispecialty clinics

Patients are seen frequently in clinic; those on targeted therapies in WHO classes III and IV, 3-monthly or more often depending on their clinical state. Multidisciplinary, multispecialist teams are usually necessary to disentangle and focus on the separate complex disease processes in associated PAH. Joint clinics with cardiologists, rheumatologists, dermatologists, and chest physicians provide breadth and depth of expertise. Even in the relatively simpler condition of IPAH, a multidisciplinary approach is required as disease diagnosis and management is complex. Important team members include:
- A physician with specialist knowledge of PH.

- A radiologist with a specialist interest in PAH, to differentiate significant lung conditions and identify CTEPH and PVOD—the latter may importantly only manifest after initiation of treatment.
- Nurse specialists to manage ongoing care and provide access to immediate specialist knowledge.
- Pharmacists with specialist knowledge of PH drugs and their interactions.
- A clinical psychologist to help with the trauma of managing a chronic often terminal illness.
- A social worker to help with the life-changing consequences of chronic disability.

The consultation

Successful and positive consultations are most likely to be achieved by friendly, interested, expert staff in comfortable, calm surroundings which allow the patient to be at ease to discuss their condition. PAH management differs from routine outpatient cardiology and chest medicine because in many countries, there are only a few specialist PAH centres with the necessary expertise and licence to prescribe and manage targeted therapies, and so the majority of patients have to travel long distances to clinic and understandably get very anxious before their consultation.

Continuity of care

Continuity of care provided by familiar faces is appreciated and valued by patients and their families and is more efficient. Patients are able to discuss their fears and concerns with expert clinicians who understand them and know their condition well. The consultation is an important component of care and is therapeutic, particularly in PAH associated with other conditions.

Patients usually attend clinic with members of their family or friends and it is important that as many as possible of the patient's social network are 'in the loop' and fully understand the clinical and management issues. The consultations are unhurried and as detailed as necessary depending on the patient.

End of life issues

As in other serious chronic conditions, great care is given to patients in the final stage of their illness. Psychosocial support, management of anxiety and depression, referral to specialist palliative care teams, counsellors, and in some cases, psychiatrists or psychologists, may be helpful. Optimum care requires sensitivity, time, and practical help which should be coordinated by the PAH multidisciplinary team.

Patients are often under shared care and seen in their local hospital and a PH centre.

Issues to be addressed in clinic include:

- Is the diagnosis secure? This is particularly important in patients referred from non-PAH centres. A variety of tests may be performed and some may need repeating. These include: blood tests, echocardiography or RHC, lung function testing, CTPA and HRCT lung scanning. Further specialist input may required from rheumatologists, respiratory physicians, hepatologists and gastroenterologists, GUCH (grown-up congenital heart disease) specialist, and cardiologists depending on the primary specialty of the physician evaluating the patient in the PH centre.
- PAH clinicians have to understand and clarify the patient's current symptoms, fears, anxieties, and areas of ignorance about PAH or other condition. Education and, when possible, reassurance of the patient and family is important.
- The patient's functional capacity, WHO class, 6MWD, and degree of disability in daily activities, have to be described and recorded.
- All other associated or unassociated medical conditions should be assessed and documented to understand their impact on the patient's life.
- Is the patient coping at home? What can be done to make their lives easier? Do they need admission to hospital for investigations or changes to their treatment? Is the patient taking the medications as prescribed? Is targeted therapy indicated? If the patient is already on targeted therapy, is the dose optimal/should another targeted therapy be added? If the patient is not on anticoagulation, are there any contraindications (POPH, previous important bleed)?
- Are there associated conditions which require treatment?
- Are there any adverse effects of treatment?
- Patients with PAH associated with CTD or other conditions are optimally managed in a joint specialist rheumatology/PAH clinic, by senior experienced staff who can address all the patient's concerns. These may include: breathlessness due to PAH, ILD, CAD, myocardial fibrosis, symptoms of CTD (gut, skin, joint, and muscle symptoms), haematological, renal, liver, and neurological problems.
- Peripheral oedema may be due to right heart failure, causing gut oedema and impaired absorption of oral diuretics, which may then need to be changed, ↑, or given intravenously.
- Peripheral oedema may also be due to an ERA or calcium antagonist, or other causes which should be explored.
- Patients who have been seen or who are under review by a surgical centre for LT or PEA are usually also seen in the surgical centre.
- Patients are often seen by non-PAH specialists in their local hospital as well as specialists in the PAH centre. This is called shared care. There are advantages of a coordinated collaborative view of these complex patients with all specialists acutely aware of duplication of tests and avoiding confusing messages and conflicting management plans. Outreach clinics are popular with patients and local specialists solve some of these problems.
- Regular close clinical monitoring of patients allows clinicians to detect changes in the condition. Deterioration may prompt

further investigations including lung function, HRCT lung scanning, echocardiography, cardiac catheterization, reconsideration of the diagnosis (has something been missed or is there a new problem? E.g. coronary heart disease, ASD, shunt, CTEPH or new PEs?

- Patients with CTD may develop complications of their primary condition (e.g. renal crisis and/or lung fibrosis in SSc, myocardial fibrosis, and heart failure).
- Potential adverse effects to treatment have to be evaluated and include: renal impairment due to diuretics or the underlying condition, LFT abnormalities or oedema or drug interactions with ERAs, intolerance to PDE-5Is, infected IV indwelling catheters used for prostanoids, painful indurated skin with subcutaneous prostanoids, bradycardia with digoxin, unsatisfactory INR levels with warfarin. A significant proportion (~10%) of patients cannot tolerate ERAs or PDE-5Is and these may need to be stopped or switched to an alternative drug.
- Psychological and social problems: most patients have some degree of depression and many are tearful and isolated. Most countries have a PAH patient association which provides practical advice and support, improving their confidence and emotional health. A large number of UK patients are brought to the PAH clinic by hospital transport. There are some logistical problems with this which impact quite heavily on some patients. The majority of patients are anxious, fearful, or terrified about their condition and its implications on their life expectancy. This is often particularly severe in young women with young children. The disease often prevents the patient and their spouse from working and this has major financial implications.
- General health issues: as with any serious illness, appetite levels are usually reduced leading to weight loss and bowel disturbances. If there is significant weight loss this may have pharmacokinetic implications.
- The prospect of palliative care should be discussed with severely ill patients.

Supportive measures

Rehabilitation and exercise

Unless PAH is severe (WHO class IV), daily physical exercise is probably beneficial, improving confidence and exercise tolerance. Patients should exercise as much as they can comfortably. Mild breathlessness is usually safe. They should stop when they get very breathless, or feel faint or get chest pain. Patients can usually exercise close to their limits safely.

- Severe PAH and right heart failure with immobility lead to cardiovascular and muscular wasting and deconditioning which further impairs effort tolerance and quality of life.
- Sudden vigorous exercise in severe PAH may trigger severe breathlessness, syncope, or near syncope and angina.
- Severely deconditioned patients should undergo supervised rehabilitation, but for most patients, regular unsupervised exercise to a level associated with only mild breathlessness should be encouraged. A simple way of achieving this is for patients to undertake home 6min walking exercises on level ground twice a day.
- Fitter patients can undertake more normal exercise programmes.
- One study of using 15 weeks of cardiorespiratory training in patients with PAH and CTEPH was found to be safe, but there was no difference in echocardiographic estimates of haemodynamics, however 6MWD and quality of life improved.

Heat and RV preload

Cutaneous vasodilatation caused by hot weather, hot baths, steam baths, and saunas should be avoided in advanced PAH because of the potential fall in RV preload and CO.

Contraception in PAH

Because of the strong association between female sex and PAH, oestrogen-containing hormone therapies are discouraged. Progesterone-only hormone therapy, e.g. medroxyprogesterone acetate and etonogestrel, is preferred for women without a history of VTE or thrombophilia. ERA therapies may reduce the efficacy of oral contraceptives.

Subcutaneous Implanon® type contraception is considered particularly suitable for patients with PAH, since this ensures consistent contraception.

The Mirena® coil may also be considered. It should be inserted in hospital by an experienced practitioner with full resuscitative equipment in high-risk women because of the risk of a vagal reaction and fall in RV preload, during insertion.

Barrier methods though safe are unreliable and should only be used as adjunctive. A combination of 2 methods can be used to reduce the risk of pregnancy.

There is no evidence base or consensus on postmenopausal therapy. Hormone replacement therapy may be used for intolerable flushing, in conjunction with oral anticoagulants.

Risks of pregnancy and contraception

Maternal mortality is 30–50% and so patients are strongly discouraged from becoming pregnant.

- Most available data was recorded prior to when effective therapies were available, and case series are now being published suggesting that maternal mortality is likely to be significantly lower.
- The standard advice remains unchanged, firstly because these case series do not represent robust evidence, secondly because the medium term outlook for PAH remains poor.
- ERAs are teratogenic and should be stopped if a patient accidentally or by choice becomes pregnant and wishes to continue with the pregnancy.
- Prostanoids seem to be tolerated, but have relaxing effects on the uterus.
- PDE inhibitors have not been shown to be safe but have not been shown to be teratogenic.

Physiological changes during normal pregnancy, labour, and delivery

There is a progressive increase in total blood volume to 145% of normal with an associated increase in LV and RVEDV. HR increases by 10–20bpm, and CO increases by 30–50% by the 2nd trimester. Systemic vasodilatation and a low-resistance utero-placental resistance result in a fall in SVR by 20–30%. Pulmonary pressure remains stable due to a similar fall in PVR because the elastic distensible pulmonary vasculature can accommodate the ↑ CO and blood volume. There are no changes in CVP or PCWP. In the supine position, the IVC is compressed by the enlarging uterus, reducing CO.

During labour, delivery, and in the postpartum period, CO increases further (up to 50% during contractions), O_2 consumption increases, and HR and systemic BP increase due to pain and anxiety. During delivery, uterine contractions lead to an autotransfusion of 300–500mL of blood. 1L of placental blood may also return to the maternal circulation on delivery, leading to an increase in CO and followed by rapid falls in HR, SVR, and CO. These changes revert to normal during the postpartum period.

Haemodynamic dangers of pregnancy in PAH

In PAH, the gradual increase in CO and HR may lead to increases in mPAP and RV afterload during pregnancy. During labour, the sudden increases in blood volume and CO lead to further increases in mPAP due to the high and fixed PVR in PAH. There is an increase in RV afterload and depending on RV function, this may cause right heart failure and decreases in CO. Most maternal deaths among PAH patients occur within the 1st month after delivery.

Termination of pregnancy

Early termination is advised for accidental pregnancy. This should be done ideally in the 1st trimester. Suction curettage under local anaesthesia is recommended.

Diagnosis of PAH during pregnancy

Maternal mortality is higher if PAH is diagnosed late and if PAH is severe.

Most CHD-PAH patients are diagnosed in childhood. IPAH may be first diagnosed in pregnancy. Features of PAH and right heart failure: fatigue, breathlessness, syncope, and ankle swelling, may be misinterpreted as features of pregnancy. Echocardiography should be performed if significant breathlessness or syncope occurs and referral to a specialist PAH centre is vital if PAH is suspected on echocardiographic findings.

Management of pregnancy in PAH

There is little evidence other than case series to guide management. For those who choose to continue with pregnancy, targeted therapies, despite the risk of teratogenicity, planned early elective delivery with close collaboration between the obstetrician, anaesthetist, and the PH team is recommended. Patients should be seen monthly and some may be admitted to hospital early during pregnancy for monitoring which should be performed perhaps monthly to check for intrauterine growth retardation which may occur in 30% of cases—particularly in babies born to mothers with antiphospholipid antibodies and SLE-PAH.

Delivery should be planned in a PH centre with full facilities to deal with complications. Incremental epidural anaesthesia is recommended

Both vaginal and Caesarean section are reasonable.

The aim for delivery is to minimize danger to the mother and baby by avoiding increases in PVR, mPAP, and right heart strain.

General measures

- Pregnant women with PAH should rest, not perform vigorous exercise or activities, and reduce IVC compression by lying on their side rather than their back.
- Diuretics may be necessary for volume overload. O_2 is given for hypoxaemia.
- Warfarin and other vitamin K antagonists are avoided and LMWH is recommended throughout pregnancy.

PAH-specific therapies

- The risk of pregnancy in PAH is lowest in the small minority of IPAH patients who respond to CCBs and whose mPAP normalize or reduce to near normal levels.
- Both nifedipine and diltiazem are safe to use during pregnancy.
- Prostanoids and PDE-5Is appear safe.
- ERAs are potent teratogens and contraindicated during pregnancy.

Lifestyle issues

Travel

Patients with PAH should travel with adequate written information on their condition and a sufficient supply of therapy.

Those on IV and targeted therapies should know the location and how to contact the closest PH centre offering quality specialized medical care.

Holidays at altitude may present particular challenges as atmospheric oxygen concentrations are reduced at around 1500m. This may lead to ↑ breathlessness, and since hypoxia is a pulmonary vasoconstrictor, this could potentially lead to RV decompensation. There is, however, no evidence that these are more than theoretical concerns. O_2 supplementation to maintain oxygen saturations at greater than 90% is generally advised, particularly for those in WHO classes III and IV.

Fitness to fly testing

Fitness to fly testing (by saturation and blood gas assessment while inspiring 15% O_2) is practised in many centres, and O_2 therapy during flights or at altitude is guided based on direct testing. Supplemental O_2 is advised for patients in WHO classes III and IV and those whose O_2 saturation is <90%. A flow rate of 2L/min will increase O_2 saturation to sea level values, though most aircraft provide 4L/min flow rates, so if there are any concerns in respect of CO_2 retention this needs to be explored.

Infection risk and vaccination

In common with other chronically ill patients, infection is poorly tolerated by PAH patients. 7% of PAH patients die from infections, mainly pneumonia. Influenza and pneumococcal vaccination are recommended.

When undertaking travel to tropical areas appropriate vaccination and prophylaxis should be undertaken.

PAH and potential problems with other drugs
- Vasoconstrictors (sympathomimetics for nasal congestion) may increase PAP.
- β-blockers, blunt increases in heart rate to compensate for reduced CO, and may cause pulmonary vasoconstriction.
- Warfarin has implications for travel since change in diet and time zones may affect INR.
- Warfarin interacts with antibiotics and agents that induce or inhibit cytochrome P450. In addition agents that promote gastrointestinal bleeding (NSAIDs) need to be used with caution.
- Using warfarin in people who may be prone to blackouts has potential risks, and any head injury should lead to consideration of the possibility of intracranial haemorrhage.

Elective surgery in patients with PAH

General anaesthetics in patients with PAH are associated with substantially ↑ risks. The risk depends on the right heart haemodynamics, and RV function and CO. Local and epidural anaesthesia are probably safer, at least in higher-risk individuals. Paradoxically, PEA for very ill patients with advanced PAH is the definitive therapy, but of course successful surgery is associated with very reduced postoperative risks.

Emergency surgery and prolonged surgery (>3h) are strongly associated with adverse outcomes. When considering surgery in patients with PAH the risk:benefit ratio assessment should recognize that there is a mortality of between 10–30% for even moderate risk procedures.

For elective procedures, a multidisciplinary approach considering the mode of anaesthesia and likely physiological consequences, the likely peri- and postoperative adverse events (e.g. gastrointestinal stasis, infection), and how to manage these, is important. Where possible, elective surgery in PAH should be done in a PAH centre or after discussion with the patient's PAH specialist. In particular the use of IV pulmonary vasodilator therapy should be considered perioperatively.

Most sedatives reduce BP and should be used with caution. Anaesthetic advice should be sought from experts dealing with PAH, e.g. those in thromboendarterectomy centres. At present it is unknown whether regional or general anaesthesia is preferred; epidural and regional or local anaesthesia are preferred.

Even minor procedures are associated with significant risk. In patients with well managed PAH, it is particularly important that PAH therapy is not interrupted, shifting to IV therapy should be considered if there is any possibility of an interruption to oral treatment.

Management of arrhythmias

Precipitating factors for arrhythmias should be sought by investigating and treating infection, electrolyte abnormalities, thyroid disorders. Lifestyle factors including alcohol, caffeine, and smoking are rare in most cases of PAH and may be more common in HIV-PAH and POPH. Patients should be asked about their use of proprietary over-the-counter drugs (sympathomimetics and cold remedies).

Ventricular arrhythmias

Compared to left heart disease and left heart failure, arrhythmias are uncommon in PAH. Ventricular tachycardia or ventricular fibrillation is only occasionally the cause of death in PAH.

Atrial arrhythmias

Atrial arrhythmias may cause sudden severe haemodynamic compromise due to right heart failure in PAH. Restoring sinus rhythm quickly is important.

Despite the potential serious increase in bosentan levels, amiodarone may need to be used for severe, haemodynamically important attacks of paroxysmal AF.

Radiofrequency ablation can be used for medically refractory, symptomatic, haemodynamically important atrial flutter and AF.

There are no RCTs comparing treatments of atrial arrhythmias in PAH and so management is tailored to the patient's clinical state and underlying condition.

Further reading

Handler C, Coghlan G. *Pulmonary arterial hypertension: the facts.* Oxford: OUP; 2010.

Chapter 32

Specific therapies for PAH

Supportive medical therapies in PAH *210*
Advanced therapies for PAH *212*
Classes of recommendations for procedures and
  treatments *218*
Drug interactions with PAH targeted therapies *219*
Combination therapy in PAH *220*
Problems in conducting PAH drug trials *222*
Surgical interventions *225*

Supportive medical therapies in PAH

Anticoagulation

Anticoagulation, usually warfarin, is recommended for most patients with PAH. The rationale is based on the high frequency of thrombotic lesions in postmortem studies, the observed prothrombotic coagulation abnormalities, abnormalities in the fibrinolytic and coagulation pathways, and endothelial abnormalities, and the general prothrombotic factors—immobility and heart failure, which increase the risk of thromboembolism. Indwelling catheters for administration of prostanoids may increase the risk of local clotting and VTE, and anticoagulation is recommended for these patients.

The evidence is *not* based on randomized trials; the evidence from registry studies, mainly on patients with IPAH, was collected before the advent of modern targeted therapies, and from single centres. The 3-year survival was 49% in anticoagulated patients and 21% in those not treated. These observations suggest that in both IPAH and aminorex-induced PAH, anticoagulation is associated with improved survival.

The results of these studies, despite their limitations, are extended to all PAH patients except those with clotting abnormalities, a risk of bleeding or a history of bleeding (gut telangiectasia in patients with SSc, CHD [risk of haemoptysis] and any other cause or potential cause of gastrointestinal/genitourinary bleeding) and POPH with oesophageal varices, or HIV with thrombocytopenia.

> The benefits of anticoagulation have to be weighed against its risks in individual patients.

Although prostaglandins partially inhibit platelet aggregation, anticoagulation is still usually recommended in patients on prostanoids, since these are often the sickest and most immobile patients, who are at further risk of thrombosis due to their *in situ* catheter.

INR levels are kept between 2–3 in the US and UK, 1.5–2.5 in Europe.

In high-risk patients, e.g. those with CTEPH, who may be at risk from further thromboembolism if they are not fully anticoagulated, LMWH is substituted for warfarin, when warfarin has to be temporarily stopped, e.g. before surgery, some invasive dental work, or repeat cardiac catheterization. Patients or their relatives can administer the LMWH.

Diuretics

Although there are no RCT data on the effects of diuretics in PAH, there is clear symptomatic benefit in those with fluid overload.

Decompensated right heart failure leads to hepatic and gastrointestinal congestion plus ascites, with abdominal discomfort and malabsorption. Diuretics may need to be given intravenously in severe right heart failure and impaired drug absorption due to an oedematous gut wall. Severe peripheral oedema leads to reduced mobility and threatens the integrity of the skin.

There is no evidence base to guide choice of diuretic. Potassium-sparing diuretics and aldosterone antagonists (spironolactone) in preventing hypokalaemia appear logical. Aldosterone antagonists may also be beneficial for myocardial fibrosis which contributes to heart failure.

Rigid fluid and salt restriction are recommended in some centres but generally not in the UK. However, a low-salt diet is advisable and patients should be told about food preparation. Ready-made meals generally contain significant amounts of salt and should be avoided or restricted. Renal function and electrolytes should be checked frequently to help avoid pre-renal failure and electrolyte disturbances.

Oxygen

In some patients with PAH due to hypoxaemia, an acute increase in arterial O_2 saturation reduces PVR. However, there is no RCT demonstrating long-term benefit. O_2 therapy is proposed to reduce dyspnoea and improves exercise capacity and survival in patients with severe hypoxic lung disease. Nocturnal supplementation in Eisenmenger's does not improve outcome.

Many patients get significant symptomatic benefit from O_2 supplementation, though effects on exercise performance are inconsistent. Even small, light 'portable' O_2 cylinders are a significant burden to weak debilitated PAH patients.

Most PAH patients have mild hypoxaemia at rest except those with CHD or pulmonary-to-systemic shunts, or a patent foramen ovale, in whom severe hypoxaemia is the norm—in the CHD population there is no evidence for benefit from oxygen supplementation and treatment is generally not recommended. Blood oxygen levels should be maintained at >8kPa for 15h a day in those with non-shunt-related hypoxaemia, based on data from the COPD population, and O_2 should be given during exercise if there is symptomatic benefit and correctable desaturation on exercise.

Antidepressants

Abnormalities of the serotonin pathway are found in PAH. There has been no trial of SSRI therapy in PAH, but because some patients are depressed, SSRIs combined with counselling and psychological support may be beneficial.

Digoxin

Digoxin, a weak inotrope in patients with heart failure, acutely improves RV function in PAH, but its long-term efficacy is unknown.

Many patients with advanced PAH have significant tachycardia. Digoxin reduces the heart rate at rest without compromising exercise heart rate and is believed to benefit some patients. It helps to control the ventricular response in patients with uncontrolled AF. A dose of 0.125–0.25mg is usually prescribed but this may need to be reduced in the elderly and those with impaired renal function.

Advanced therapies for PAH

Recent therapeutic advances in PAH treatment

20 years ago the only medical therapies with an evidence base were CCBs and warfarin. Since then, the advances in our understanding of the pathogenesis of PAH have led to new therapies, targeting these pathophysiological and molecular abnormalities.

PAH is rare and it is difficult recruiting sufficient numbers of patients into RCTs. Most RCTs in PAH have included the common types of PAH: idiopathic, heritable, and associated with anorexigens and toxins, CTDs, CHD, and HIV. Few patients with other types of PAH have been studied. A small number of trials have enrolled patients with a single aetiology of PAH (e.g. CTD, Eisenmenger's syndrome, and HIV). Data on safety, efficacy, and outcomes from treatments for one type of PAH may not apply to other types of PAH although in clinical practice, it is assumed that all types of PAH respond similarly.

Rationale for early diagnosis and treatment

Information about survival with current PAH-targeted therapies comes from registry data and not long-term RCTs. It appears that survival after 3–5 years of treatment has improved. Meta-analysis of RCTs of all therapies shows that at 14 weeks, mortality has improved by 40%. Early diagnosis and treatment of PAH is therefore important.

Pathogenetic pathways targeted by therapies

All current licensed therapies address 3 pathways:
- The endothelin pathway using endothelin receptor blocking agents.
- The NO pathway using PDE-5Is.
- The prostacyclin pathway using prostanoids.

Using more than one therapy to target more than one pathway, ('combination therapy') becomes necessary and appears sensible in the majority of patients as their disease progresses, although the evidence base for this approach is still weak.

PAH is a progressive condition and patients deteriorate despite therapy. Frequent monitoring and evaluation of patients clinically and haemodynamically, and using other tests is necessary so that changes in treatment can be made.

Specific therapies

Calcium channel blockers in vasodilator positive patients
- Vasoconstriction plays a major role in PAH and CCBs were shown 20 years ago to be effective in some patients.
- CCBs are not recommended in PVOD/PCH because of the risk of pulmonary oedema. This risk is also present in CTD-PAH.
- CCBs should be prescribed only to patients with a positive acute vasoreactivity response because of the risk of hypotension without a fall in PVR.
- Repeat right heart catheterization is the most accurate method to confirm continued response to CCBs. Only 6% of IPAH patients

respond long term. Therefore, all acute responders should be carefully monitored in specialist centres to identify and switch treatment in those who deteriorate. Haemodynamic deterioration is most accurately determined by cardiac catheterization and in our centre, this is done after 3 months and annually.
- There is evidence of benefit for high-dose nifedipine (120–240mg/d), amlodipine (20mg/d), and diltiazem (240–720mg/d) in acute responders. The dose is limited by side effects (peripheral oedema, hypotension, headaches, etc.).
- Diltiazem is recommended in the setting of tachycardia. Those who have near normalization of pressures at 3 months have a near normal 5-year survival. Verapamil is not recommended because it has significantly greater negative inotropic effects.
- Long-term vasodilators rarely benefit SSc-PAH and other associated types of PAH.
- Common side effects of dihydropyridine CCBs are ankle swelling— which is not usually severe and easily treated with low-dose diuretics— postural hypotension, and flushing.

Intravenous epoprostenol
- Epoprostenol is a synthetic prostacyclin in powder form. It is dissolved in alkaline fluid. Because it has a half-life of only 3–5min it is administered as a continuous infusion through a tunnelled line into the SVC.
- In 3 unblinded, short-term RCTs in IPAH and SSC-PAH, it improved symptoms, exercise tolerance, and haemodynamics by reducing PVR by 25% and increasing CO by 15%. In one trial a benefit in mortality was found, though the trial was not powered for this outcome.
- Registry data suggest that epoprostenol improves survival and well-being in IPAH and associated PAH.
- Treatment is initiated at low doses (2–4ng/kg/min) and usually ↑ toward around 20ng/kg/min over 3 months. Dose increases are limited by side-effects. Higher doses (20–40ng/kg/min) are often used, but it is unclear whether the need for higher doses is evidence of treatment failure or tachyphylaxis.
- Abrupt cessation of epoprostenol may lead to rebound PH with decompensation, heart failure and death. Systems must be in place to ensure continuous delivery and patients should have written instructions to carry with them with contact numbers of their specialist centre and a senior clinician familiar with their case. It is not unusual for these sick patients to be admitted to a non-expert centre, for a non-associated condition or deterioration in right heart failure, to be found to be 'hypotensive' and the epoprostenol is stopped without consultation with the PAH centre.
- Septicaemia due to line infection is the 2nd major threat. Strict guidelines for insertion and management of catheters must be in place, with a comprehensive educational programme to ensure that patient self-management is optimal and that all their medical attendants are aware of what to look for and how this potentially very serious complication is managed.
- Sepsis should always be considered in the event of acute deterioration.

Iloprost

- Iloprost is a stable prostacyclin analogue available as inhaled and IV forms.
- Only the inhaled form has been shown in RCTs improve exercise tolerance, symptoms, PVR, and clinical events when administered 6–9 times daily in IPAH and CTEPH.
- Side effects of inhaled iloprost include flushing and jaw pain.
- Some patients find the preparation and administration of inhaled iloprost too time consuming and practically difficult.
- IV iloprost has shown similar exercise performance and haemodynamic benefits as epoprostenol in open-label studies.

Treprostinil

- Treprostinil is a stable analogue of epoprostenol. Inhaled, intravenous, subcutaneous and oral forms have been developed. The inhaled and oral forms have yet to gain licences.
- Subcutaneous administration was shown to improve exercise performance, haemodynamics, and symptoms in a large RCT. However, significant local site discomfort restricted widespread use. Registry data suggest that those who can tolerate long-term therapy have improved survival associated with sustained exercise benefit.
- Inhaled treprostinil when added on to an ERA or sildenafil has been shown to improve exercise capacity and symptoms when administered 4 times daily.
- There is no evidence that oral treprostinil is superior to placebo. A further study is underway.
- IV treprostinil has been evaluated in one double blind trial and found superior to placebo. Unfortunately the trial was marred by a high complication rate which may have reduced the pharmacological effect.

Beraprost

An oral stable analogue of prostacyclin that is available in Japan. It shares the common prostanoid side effects.

Endothelin and endothelin receptor antagonists

- PAH is associated with activation of the endothelin (ET) system with ↑ levels of ET.
- ET levels are associated with prognosis. ET levels are also ↑ in atherosclerosis, systemic hypertension, and heart failure.
- The human ET family consists of three 21-amino acid isopeptides: ET-1, ET-2, ET-3. Only ET-1 is important in controlling vascular tone.
- ET is released from endothelial cells which line blood vessels, and is a vasoconstrictor, is profibrotic and proinflammatory, and is a mitogen, promoting hypertrophy and hyperplasia.
- ET also stimulates the production of NO, prostacyclins, and platelet-activating factors which modulate ET effects.

Endothelin receptors

ET-1 exerts effects through 2 receptor subtypes: ET-$_A$ and ET-$_B$. ET-$_A$ receptors are located on SMCs and fibroblasts. ET-$_B$ receptors are localized on endothelial cells, SMCs, and fibroblasts. Physiologically, the receptor types have opposing actions. Activation of ET-$_A$ mediates vaso-constriction, proliferation, hypertrophy, cell migration, and fibrosis. ET-$_B$ receptors on the endothelial cells mediate the clearance of circulating ET-1 in the lungs, kidney, and liver and release of vasodilators and anti-proliferative substances, NO, and prostacyclin resulting in vasodilatation. In theory, selective ET-$_A$ with resulting vasodilatation should be advanta-geous but this has not been shown clinically. There appears to be no clini-cally important difference between selective and non-selective ERAs.

Endothelin receptor antagonists

There have been no head-to-head studies comparing the efficacy or safety of the 2 available ERAs. They are considered to have similar efficacy and there is no evidence that one is superior or inferior in any type of PAH.

The choice of ERA is based on the specialist's individual experience and interpretation of the trials.

Both available ERAs have been shown in double-blind, placebo-controlled studies conducted over 16 weeks to:
- Improve 6MWD by around 36m.
- Improve functional class.
- Improve haemodynamics.
- Slow down the rate of deterioration measured by an increase in the time to clinical worsening.
- Persistence of benefit for at least 1 year (registry data).

Bosentan and ambrisentan are licensed in Europe for WHO classes II, III, and IV and in classes III and IV in the UK.

The most serious adverse effect of ERAs is liver toxicity, which is clinically important when the transaminases are >3× upper limit of normal. This is perhaps least likely with ambrisentan but with all ERAs, is usually reversible, and dose dependent. All patients on ERAs must have monthly LFTs; the drug may need to be discontinued if for any reason this is not done.

ERAs and CTD-PAH

There are no long-term RCTs showing a benefit of ERAs in CTD-PAH but registry data suggested that current treatment strategies including bosentan were superior to survival before the availability of oral agents. Sitaxsentan (which has been voluntarily withdrawn) was shown to be at least as good in a 1-year extension of the STRIDE 2 trial. Registry data on ambrisentan showed similar survival of CTD-PAH as IPAH. These data support ERA therapy as 1st-line treatment in SSc-PAH although there is no evidence that ERAs are superior to other therapies.

Bosentan

- Bosentan is an oral dual endothelin receptor antagonist. It is also licensed for patients in WHO-II and with CHD and Eisenmenger's syndrome.
- Dosage is started at 62.5mg twice daily and ↑ to 125mg twice daily after 1 month if there are no LFT derangements or other important adverse effects. Registry data suggest that survival is ↑ at least in adults with IPAH.

- LFT abnormalities occur in around 10% of patients. Peripheral oedema is not uncommon. Drug–drug interactions are common with bosentan because of its induction of CYP3A4 and CYP2C9. Haemoglobin levels may fall slightly.

Sitaxsentan

- Sitaxsentan was withdrawn from all clinical use in 2010 due to cases of unpredictable serious liver injury. This illustrates the potential for serious adverse effects from this group of drugs and the importance of close supervision and monitoring of patients including monthly LFTs.
- Sitaxsentan was an orally active selective ET-$_A$ inhibitor. Dosage was 100mg once daily.
- Post-marketing surveillance studies and clinical trials showed reversible LFT abnormalities in 4% of patients. Drug–drug interactions were less frequent than with bosentan.

Ambrisentan

Ambrisentan mainly blocks ET-$_A$ receptors. Drug–drug interactions are less frequent compared to the other 2 ERAs. LFT abnormalities occur in 2% of patients. Peripheral oedema is comparatively uncommon. Dosage is either 5mg or 10mg once daily. as a dose response has been demonstrated for this agent.

Phosphodiesterase-5 inhibitors

NO deficiency has been documented in PAH, and inhaled NO is a powerful vasodilator in this condition, but difficult to administer long term. PDE-5 is abundant in the lung and degrades cGMP (cyclic guanosine monophosphate), reducing NO production. Inhibitors of PDE-5 increase NO bioavailability with vasodilating and antiproliferative effects.

There is no evidence that PDE-5Is are either superior or inferior to ERAs.

Sildenafil

Sildenafil is an orally active PDE-5I. It is licensed for use at 20mg three times daily based on the SUPER trial in PAH, where beneficial effects on symptoms, exercise capacity, and haemodynamics were shown at 12 weeks. In the UK the dose is usually ↑ to 50 mg three times daily after 1 month. Maximum effects occur 60min after administration.

Post hoc analysis suggest equivalent efficacy in the CTD population. Sildenafil 80mg three times daily added to epoprostenol IV has been shown to improve exercise capacity and delay clinical worsening, and reduce death rate. An IV preparation of sildenafil has been developed.

Side effects of sildenafil relate to vasodilation and include nasal congestion, occasionally nose bleeds, flushing, and headaches. A rare but important side effect is NION (non-ischaemic optic neuropathy) which can cause loss of vision.

Drug interactions of note are profound hypotension with nitrates and nicorandil (important in a population prone to angina) and inhibition of sildenafil metabolism by protease inhibitors. If used with bosentan, sildenafil levels are reduced and bosentan levels ↑ due to interaction via cytochrome P450 3A4. Higher doses of sildenafil should be considered if bosentan is also prescribed.

Tadalafil

Tadalafil is a once-daily oral PDE-5I licensed in some countries at 40mg/d. In a large trial in PAH, tadalafil improved exercise performance, symptoms, and haemodynamics. At 40mg/d it delays time to clinical worsening. Maximum effects occur after 90min.

Additive benefit to background bosentan was also demonstrated as nearly half the patients were on this background therapy in the trial.

The side effect profile is similar to sildenafil. Fewer drug–drug interactions occur, but the interaction with nicorandil and nitrates is universal with this group of drugs.

Dose–response characteristics of specific PAH drugs

Ambrisentan is the only ERA that has been shown to have a dose–response curve (greater efficacy at 10mg than at 5mg). Neither bosentan nor sitaxsentan show ↑ efficacy with increasing dosage.

PDE-5Is appear to have a flat dose responses. Sildenafil shows a flat dose response curve between 20–80mg three times daily—at least in terms of walking distance. Tadalafil has only one proven dose of 40mg/d.

By contrast prostanoids, epoprostenol, and treprostinil, show clear dose responses, but dose escalation is generally limited by side effects. Experience with IV epoprostenol over the last 2 decades has shown that in order to maintain efficacy, the dose has to be ↑ regularly. Despite big doses, published registries of patients treated with ambulatory epoprostenol show only a 63% 3-year survival, much better than without treatment, but still very poor, disappointing, and demoralizing for a young population. Even for less sick patients receiving initial oral therapy (mainly ERA) the 3-year survival is <80%. The situation is significantly worse for patients with scleroderma-associated PAH with a 3-year survival in the UK registry 2001–2006 of only 47%.

Prostanoids

- Prostacyclin (epoprostenol, PGI_2) is produced mainly by vascular endothelial cells, it induces vasodilation, inhibits platelet aggregation, and has cytoprotective and antiproliferative effects. It inhibits SMC growth *in vitro*.
- Prostacyclin synthetase activity is reduced in the PAs of patients with PAH, and this is thought to promote vasoconstriction.
- Side effects are dose dependent and are common to all prostanoids. The common side effects include flushing, headache, diarrhoea, jaw pain, and leg pain.

Classes of recommendations for procedures and treatments

- *Class I:* evidence and/or general agreement that a given treatment or procedure is beneficial, useful, and effective
- *Class II:* conflicting opinion on the usefulness/efficacy of the treatment or procedure
- *Class IIa:* weight of evidence in favour of usefulness/efficacy
- *Class IIb:* usefulness/efficacy is less well established by evidence/opinion
- *Class III:* evidence or general agreement that the treatment or procedure is not effective/useful and in some cases may be harmful

Level of evidence of efficacy of PAH-targeted therapies

- *A* Data from multiple RCTs or meta-analyses
- *B* Data from a single RCT or large non-randomized studies
- *C* Consensus of opinion of the experts and/or small studies, retrospective studies, registries

Also see Table 32.1.

Table 32.1 Levels of evidence for PAH-specific therapies and other treatments for PAH according to WHO functional class

Drug or procedure	FCII	FCIII	FCIV
CCBs	I-C[a]	I-C[a]	–
Ambrisentan	I-A	I-A	IIa-C
Bosentan	I-A	I-A	IIa-C
Sildenafil	I-A	I-A	IIa-C
Tadalafil[b]		IIb-B	–
Epoprostenol IV	–	I-A	I-A
Iloprost inhaled	–	I-A	IIa-C
Iloprost IV	–	IIa-C	IIa-C
Trepostinil SC	–	I-B	IIa-C
Trepostinil IV	–	IIa-C	IIa-C
Trepostinil inhaled[b]	–	I-B	IIa-C
Initial combination Rx	–	–	IIa-C
Sequential combination Rx	IIa-C	IIa-B	IIa-B
Balloon atrial septostomy	–	I-C	I-C
Lung Tx	–	I-C	I-C

[a]Only in responders to acute vasoreactivity tests

I for idiopathic PAH, heritable PAH, and PAH due to anorexigens; IIa for APAH conditions

[b]Under regulatory review in the European Union

CCBs, calcium channel blockers; FC, WHO functional class; Lung Tx, lung transplantation.

Drug interactions with PAH targeted therapies

Bosentan is an inducer of cytochrome P450 isoenzymes CYP3A4 and CYP2C9. Plasma concentrations of drugs metabolized by these isoenzymes will be reduced when given with bosentan. Bosentan is also metabolized by these enzymes so their inhibition may increase the plasma concentration of bosentan.

A potent CYP2C9 inhibitor (e.g. amiodarone or fluconazole), combined with a potent CYP3A4 inhibitor (e.g. ketoconazole or ritonavir) and bosentan may cause a significant increase in bosentan levels; this combination is contraindicated.

Sildenafil is metabolized by cytochrome P450 isoenzymes CYP3A4 and CYP2CP. There is an increase in sildenafil levels and reduced clearance with CYP3A4 substrates. CYP3A4 inducers, e.g. carbamazepine, phenytoin, phenobarbital, rifampicin, and St John's wort may significantly lower sildenafil levels. Sildenafil levels are modestly ↑ by fresh grapefruit juice, a weak inhibitor of CYP3A4. Also see Table 32.2.

Table 32.2 Potential drug interactions with PAH-targeted therapies

Therapy	Drug	Interaction
Ambrisentan	Cyclosporine	Caution required
	Ketoconazole	
Bosentan	Sildenafil	S ↓ 50% B ↑ 50%
	Cyclosporine	Cyclosporine ↓ 50%. B ↑ x4.*
Bosentan	Erythromycin	B ↑↑
	Ketoconazole	B ↑ x2
Bosentan	Glibenclamide	Aminotransferase ↑. ↓ effect of glib*
Bosentan	Fluconazole	B ↑↑*
	Amiodarone	
Bosentan	Rifampicin	B ↓ 58%
	Phenytoin	
Bosentan	Statins	Statin levels d 50%. Check lipids
Bosentan	OC	Hormone levels ↓. OC unreliable
Bosentan	Warfarin	Warfarin ↓. Check INR
Sildenafil	Bosentan	Sildenafil ↓ 50%. Bosentan ↓ 50%
Sildenafil	Statins	Statin ↑. Sildenafil ↑. Rhabdomyolysis
Sildenafil	HIV protease inhibitors	Sildenafil ↑↑
Sildenafil	Phenytoin	Sildenafil ↓
Sildenafil	Erythromycin	Sildenafil ↑↑
PDE-5I	Nitrates	BP ↓↓↓↓
	Nicorandil	

*Combination contraindicated. ↑, levels increase; ↑↑, levels increase a lot; ↓, levels decrease; BP↓↓, profound hypotension; OC, oral contraceptive; PDE-5I, phosphodiesterase-5 inhibitor.

Combination therapy in PAH

What is combination therapy?

Any combination of PAH specific treatments (e.g. ERAs, PDE-5Is, prostanoids, and novel drugs) but excluding background therapies. CCBs are also excluded from the definition of combination therapy because in the small minority of patients where they are effective, the pulmonary pressure falls without the need for additional PAH specific medication.

Possible dual combinations are:
- ERA +PDE-5I.
- ERA + prostanoid.
- PDE-5I + prostanoid.
- All 3 classes combined.
- Any one of these listed plus a novel investigational drug.

Rationale for combination therapy

PAH is progressive. Any single therapy may stabilize the condition or even improve it for a while, but there is no cure.

As in other chronic disease states, e.g. systemic hypertension, adding in a drug from a different class which acts on a different pathogenetic pathway, might result in improvement. This may be additive or synergistic.

Registry data from small patient numbers suggest combination therapy may help stabilize in the short-term.

There is no evidence, however, from long-term RCTs that combination therapy improves survival over monotherapy. Nevertheless, combination therapy is common practice in PAH centres worldwide. There are major cost constraints which restrict this relatively new practice.

Safety of combination therapy

Clinically significant drug interactions between PAH specific drugs are rare and combination therapy appears to be safe.

The lack of good evidence from large long-term RCTs that combination therapy is cost-effective and worthwhile restricts its use to sick patients with very advanced PAH and heart failure.

Does combination therapy work?

There have been only a few randomized trials of combination therapies in PAH, conducted over a short period of time, some showing significant but clinically small improvements in 6MWD and time to clinical worsening and, in one case, mortality. Combination therapy yields an average 20–25m improvement in 6MWD when compared to monotherapy plus placebo. This is less than the improvement in walking distance with monotherapy when compared to placebo (approximately 45m net benefit). The effects of combination therapy on the time to clinical worsening are variable. Of the 4 large trials completed to date, one (Freedom) was entirely negative due to dosing issues and 2 of the 3 positive trials showed major benefit in terms of delaying clinical worsening, including one showing an improvement in mortality. On balance the data suggest that the benefit of combination therapy is clear but more in terms of stabilization rather than improvement. Further longer-term trials are ongoing.

Goal directed therapy

The availability of multiple therapies that can be used in combination raises the prospect of increasing treatment until an optimal outcome has been achieved. The complexity of advanced therapies such as IV prostanoids, requires that a balanced approach be taken. The ESC/ERS guidelines (2009) recommend that patients are reassessed periodically to ensure that a 'stable and satisfactory' outcome is achieved. The parameters chosen (shown in Table 32.3) are those that have provide independent prognostic information.

Table 32.3 Parameters with established importance for assessing disease severity, stability and prognosis in PAH (adapted from McLaughlin and McGoon)

Better prognosis	Determinants of prognosis	Worse prognosis
No	Clinical evidence of RV failure	Yes
Slow	Rate of progression of symptoms	Rapid
No	Syncope	Yes
I, II	WHO-FC	IV
Longer (>500 m)[a]	6MWT	Shorter (<300 m)
Peak O_2 consumption >15 mL/min/kg	Cardio-pulmonary exercise testing	Peak O_2 consumption <12 mL/min/kg
Normal or near-normal	BNP/NT-proBNP plasma levels	Very elevated and rising
No pericardial effusion TAPSE[b] >2.0 cm	Echocardiographic findings[b]	Pericardial effusion TAPSE[b] <1.5 cm
RAP <8 mmHg and CI ≥2.5 L/min/m^2	Haemodynamics	RAP >15 mmHG or CI ≤2.0 L/min/m^2

[a]Depending on age.

[b]TAPSE and pericardial effusion have been selected because they can be measured in the majority of the patients.

BNP = brain natriuretic peptide; CI = cardiac index; 6MWT = 6-minute walking test; RAP = right atrial pressure; TAPSE = tricuspid annular plane systolic excursion; WHO-FC = WHO functional class.

Problems in conducting PAH drug trials

There are several major practical problems in conducting trials in a rare, complex, and serious disease.

- It is not easy to ensure uniform standards of clinical care in international multicentre trials which are necessary to recruit adequate numbers of suitable patients.
- It is no longer considered ethical in having a placebo arm in PAH trials.
- The trial duration should be long enough to draw conclusions about long-term safety and efficacy.
- The choice of end-points should allow clear interpretation about survival and quality of life, the 2 main issues of interest to patients and their families.
- End-points should reflect the underlying disease state.

Limitations of PAH trials

From 1995–2009, 26 trials of PAH specific drugs were performed.

- Most of the PAH trials have used endpoints that were practical and met licensing requirements rather than answering the fundamental clinical questions.
- They do not include outcomes beyond those necessary for drug approval.
- The mean duration of trials was only 14 weeks.
- None of the 26 trials used survival as the primary end-point of efficacy and so it is difficult to draw conclusions about long-term effects of the drugs.
- There have been no 'head-to-head' comparisons. Therefore, it is not known if any one drug is superior to another within its class or to another from a different class.
- The trials have almost always been sponsored by the pharmaceutical industry, which has been instrumental in their design, conduct, data analysis, and publication.
- Patients with advanced lung involvement (FVC <60%) have been excluded from the pivotal trials and so it is not known if PAH-targeted treatments are effective in patients with lung involvement. Trials of ERAs in lung fibrosis have been negative.

Interpretation of exercise endpoints

6MWD is the most commonly used end-point in PAH trials. Although it is easy and cheap to measure, interpretation of its diagnostic and prognostic value is complicated by threshold effects. While those with an excellent 6MWD have a good prognosis either before or when measured on therapy, modest changes in 6MWD while associated with improved quality of life, have not been found to predict improved prognosis.

'Warm up' exercise tests are used in trials of drugs for angina to unmask a possible 'training effect' due to familiarization with the test and increasing confidence. Warm-up 6MWTs have not been part of PAH trials. If there is a significant 'training effect' in these patients, then this would complicate interpretation of improvements in 6MWD observed in PAH trials. Rehabilitation and exercise training have been shown to increase exercise capacity, and quality of life in severe chronic left heart failure, and also in PAH, independent of drug therapy.

Meta-analyses of PAH drug trials: survival

The pooled effect of all treatments strategies shows a significant reduction of 40% in all-cause mortality after a mean treatment duration of 14 weeks. However, this cumulative effect is derived by combining 3 classes of therapies that have different mechanisms of action. The benefits were confined only to patients with advanced disease for 16 weeks, regardless of which class of drug is used.

The improved survival bore no relationship with the change in 6MWD.

Combination therapies

There is also no convincing evidence that combination therapy offers a survival benefit over monotherapy and side effects may be more frequent.

RCTs of combination therapies with current drugs have shown modest improvements of only 15–25m in 6MWD, compared to 35–55m in monotherapy trials.

Long-term survival data

Meta-analyses have been used to demonstrate a 43% reduction in mortality compared to placebo. This mortality reduction is derived from 3 trials: the initial epoprostenol trials and the combination add-on trial of sildenafil to background epoprostenol, which included the sickest patients.

Long-term data on targeted therapies is derived largely from observational registry data and so conclusions are less robust than from RCTs. Current treatments may slow down progression of disease but mortality remains high. The long-term benefits of vasodilators are uncertain.

Future directions and experimental drugs

- While the current generation of drugs has revolutionized the management of PAH, patients still generally die prematurely and for most, their quality of life is poor.
- ↑ understanding of the pathobiology of PAH has revealed other pathways to explore.
- The most efficient way to test new drugs, and combination therapies, is through multicentre RCTs with relevant and meaningful long-term endpoints. Current phase III trials exploring ways to manipulate the pathways believed to be relevant in the pathogenesis of PAH and cellular proliferation include:
  - Tyrosine kinase inhibitors (imatinib has just completed a successful trial in advanced PAH)
  - Dual tissular ERA inhibition
  - Guanylate cyclase stimulators
  - VGEF inhibitors
  - Activators of cGMP
  - NO-dependent stimulators
  - Inhaled vasoactive intestinal peptide
  - Stem cell therapy
  - Selective PPAR stimulators
  - Serotonin antagonists.
- Rho-kinase inhibitors.

Future study designs and endpoints

It is now recognized that short (3–4 months) RCTs using 6MWD as the primary end-point of 6MWD are inadequate. Future trials will focus on time to clinical worsening or 'overall clinical benefit' studies and this would be accepted by the regulatory agencies. The problems with this approach include:

- Objective and uniform definition of this composite end-point.
- The sample size.
- Duration of the study, which can be either pre-specified or based on the number of observed events.
- International variations in clinical care.

Future trials need to use clinically relevant reproducible end-points which reflect the underlying disease state.

Trial duration should be long enough to enable conclusions to be drawn about long-term efficacy and safety.

Surgical interventions

Atrial septostomy

Atrial septostomy has been performed only rarely; 223 cases have been reported, mainly in women with IPAH. It has a high mortality because it is performed as a palliative procedure for end-stage PAH with intractable low output heart failure, and syncope. Acceptably low mortality depends on careful patient selection and the expertise and experience of the operator and the centre.

Indications

Baseline oxygenation should be >90% on room air, the haematocrit >35% and LV function should be normal to avoid pulmonary oedema at septostomy.

Contraindications

AS is contraindicated if the mRAP >20mmHg, O_2 saturation <80% on room air, and in patients with impending death on life support.

Rationale

An interatrial defect appears to improve survival in patients with Eisenmenger's syndrome and IPAH patients. Creating a right-to-left shunt to decompress the RA and RV, may improve systemic output and may improve survival in advanced PAH. The ↑ flow to the LV unloads the RA and RV, increases LV preload and CO, and despite arterial O_2 desaturation, improves O_2 transport and decreases sympathetic hyperactivity.

Technique

- The procedure was originally performed using blade balloon atrial septostomy but is now done using graded balloon dilatation atrial septostomy, which gives more control over the size of the septostomy. It can be done in any type of PAH.
- O_2 is given during and after the procedure, packed cells and erythropoietin have been used to increase O_2 delivery.

Survival

- Of the patients who survived atrial septostomy and had repeat RHC, there was an improvement in CO and a lower mRAP at a mean of 2 years after the procedure.
- A mean survival of 2 years after atrial septostomy suggests that the procedure had been done in relatively low-risk patients who were not 'end-stage'. There is no evidence that it improves long-term survival.
- Of the 186 survivors, 163 (87%) patients improved and 23 (12%) did not. 31 (16%) of the patients survived to receive transplantation. Mortality at 24h is 7%, and 15% at 1 month, mainly due to hypoxaemia.
- Symptoms and signs of RV failure may be improved in the short term. Spontaneous closure of the hole occurs in 12% of patients for unknown reasons but the procedure can be repeated.

Role of atrial septostomy in management of end-stage PAH
The place of atrial septostomy in the management remains unclear as there have been no prospective controlled studies looking at long-term outcomes in similar patient groups randomized to either atrial septostomy or conventional medical treatment.

Atrial septostomy is done as a palliative or bridging procedure prior to transplantation in patients with end-stage PAH after maximal medical therapies have failed.

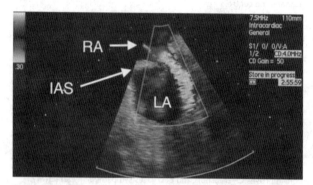

Fig. 32.1 (Also see Colour plate 5.) Intracardiac echocardiography with colour flow Doppler. A 1cm defect has been created in the intra-atrial septum (IAS), because right atrial (RA) pressure significantly exceeds left atrial (LA) pressure right-to-left flow is seen from a probe placed in the right atrium. This offloads the right ventricle while improving left ventricular filling at a cost of moderate desaturation.

Transplantation
- LT is indicated for end-stage PAH not curable by any medical therapy or conservative procedure.
- Haemodynamic criteria for LT include: mRAP >12mmHg, mPAP >60mmHg, CI <2.2L/min/m².
- Compared to liver, kidney, or heart transplantation, LT is performed rarely, mainly because of a shortage of donor lungs.
- Exclusion criteria are: age >65; respiratory failure; malignancies; other life-threatening diseases; oesophageal reflux which is common in SSc because of the risk of aspiration and damage to the transplanted lungs; phrenic nerve paralysis; mechanical respiratory paralysis.
- LT candidates are generally in WHO classes III or IV and have a life expectancy of <1 year.

Types of transplantation
Transplantation should be delayed until it offers a survival advantage over medical treatment. LT cannot be done on demand or planned because of donor lung availability. Patients on a waiting list for LT can deteriorate quite quickly with severe right heart failure and a fall in CO precipitating mulitorgan failure.

All types of LT can reduce or normalize PVR.

Double lung transplantation and heart–lung transplantation are the usual procedures performed in PAH because of the frequent V/Q mismatch observed after single LT. The donor lungs must be of good quality because of the problems in perioperative management and the susceptibility of the donor lung to infection. LT is performed under cardiopulmonary bypass.

Double LT is more commonly performed for PAH although the perioperative mortality rates, mainly due to infection and acute rejection, are higher than for single lung transplants. Later rejection is due to bronchiolitis obliterans.

Heart–lung transplantation
The procedure is relatively simple using a median sternotomy. 2 lungs and the heart are transplanted in 1 stage. It is reserved for patients who need both heart and lungs and so, apart from patients with complex CHD, is not usually required for PAH patients. Severe right heart impairment is not a contraindication to LT because RV function usually improves after LT. The donor heart should be normal avoiding left heart dysfunction.

Single-lung transplantation
This is a relatively simple operation, performed via a posterolateral thoracotomy. Only 1 lung is needed. Severe V/Q mismatch is a problem in PAH and associated with postoperative complications: reperfusion oedema, infection, rejection, which occur because the lower PVR in the normal transplanted lung allows comparatively greater perfusion. There is no difference in ventilation between the native and donor lungs.

Survival and outcomes are inferior to bilateral sequential lung transplantation or heart-lung transplantation.

Complications of lung transplantation and post-transplant immunosuppressive treatment
- Primary graft dysfunction (ischaemia reperfusion injury).
- Diaphragmatic dysfunction/paralysis.
- Vocal cord paresis.
- Chylothorax.
- Dehiscence of stricture of airway.
- Rejection—hyperacute, acute, or chronic (bronchiolitis obliterans) and respiratory failure.
- Infection associated to lifelong immunosuppression:
- Bacterial (*Staphylococcus aureus*, *Pseudomonas aeroginosa*).
- Viral (CMV and others).
- Fungal (*Aspergillus* species).
- Neoplasms: lymphomas, skin, other organs.
- Cardiovascular: systemic hypertension, air embolism, arrhythmias.
- Gastrointestinal reflux.
- Renal: calcineurin inhibitor (cyclosporine, tacrolimus) nephropathy.
- Neurological: seizures.
- Musculoskeletal: steroid myopathy, rhabdomyolysis (cyclosporine + statin).
- Osteopenia/osteoporosis.

- Avascular necrosis of hip.
- Metabolic: obesity, diabetes mellitus, hypercholesterolaemia.
- Haematological: anaemia, leucopenia, thrombocytopenia.

Survival

The postoperative survival in lung and heart–lung transplants is 80%, Overall 5- and 10-year survival rates are 49% and 36% respectively.

Index

A

activin receptor-like kinase type 1 (*ALK1*) 62, 63, 163
acute chest crisis 113
acute coronary syndromes 141
acute pulmonary embolism (PE) 67, 134, 137–145
anticoagulants, new 143
anticoagulation, long-term and venous thromboembolism (VTE) 144
anticoagulation and thrombolysis 141–2
arterial blood gas analysis 138
biomarkers (troponins and brain natriuretic peptide) 139
chest X-ray (CXR) 138
clinical decision rules 138
clinical features 138
clinical features of post-thrombotic syndrome (PTS) 144
compression stockings and post-thrombotic syndrome (PTS) 144
computed tomography of pulmonary arteries (CTPA) 140
deep vein thrombosis (DVT) 144
diagnosis and investigations 167
echocardiography (transthoracic and transoesophageal) 139
electrocardiogram (ECG) 138
phlegmasia cerulea dolens 145
pregnancy and venous thromboembolism (VTE) 145
prevention 144
pulmonary embolectomy 142
screening 144
thrombolytic therapy for deep vein thrombosis (DVT) 141
treatment 142
treatment of deep vein thrombosis (DVT) 141

vena caval interruption 142
ventilation perfusion scanning 140
warfarin 143
advanced lung disease 34
advanced therapies 212
ambrisentan 216
beraprost 214
bosentan 215
calcium channel blockers in vasodilator positive patients 212
early diagnosis and treatment rationale 212
endothelin receptor antagonists 215
endothelin receptor antagonists and connective tissue disease 215
endothelin receptors 214
epoprostenol 213
iloprost 214
pathogenetic pathways 212
phosphodiesterase-5 inhibitors 216
prostanoids 217
sitaxentan 216
therapeutic advances, recent 212
treprostinil 214
adventitia 40
aims of treatment 198
aldosterone antagonists 211
ambrisentan 215–18
drug interactions 219
human immunodeficiency virus (HIV) 90
aminorex 5, 72, 210
aminotransferase 219
amiodarone 208, 219
amlodipine 194, 212
amphetamines 72
anaemias see chronic haemolytic anaemias
anaesthesia 207
analgesics 83, 112
angiography, coronary 186
anorexigens 20, 70, 194, 212
antibiotics 112–13
anticoagulation 141, 143, 212
acute pulmonary embolism (PE) 142

chronic thromboembolic pulmonary hypertension (CTEPH) 148, 150
deep vein thrombosis (DVT) and pulmonary embolism (PE) 144
and hormone replacement therapy 203
lupus 43
portopulmonary hypertension (POPH) 96
venous thromboembolism (VTE) 144
antidepressants 211
anti-inflammatory drugs 129
antinuclear antibodies (ANA) 76–7
antiphospholipid antibodies 43, 205
antiphospholipid syndrome (APS) 82
anti-RNP (ribonuclear protein) antibody 76
anti-tumour necrosis factor (TNF) 86
aortic and mitral valve disease 67
apixaban 148
aplastic crisis 112
appetite suppressants 66, 72
Argatroban (Argatroban®) 143
arrhythmias, atrial 208
arrhythmias, ventricular 208
arterial lesions 26
arthralgia and skin rashes 83
associated conditions 75–86
dermatomyositis 76, 86
polymyositis 76, 86
Sjögren's syndrome 76, 86
see also connective tissue disease; systemic sclerosis/scleroderma; systemic lupus erythematosus
atherosclerosis 84
atrial septal defects (ASDs) 67, 100
atrial septostomy 225
azathioprine 80, 83–4, 129

B

beraprost 214
beta-blockers 96, 206
biomarkers (troponins and brain natriuretic peptide) 139, 163
bivalirudin (Angiomax®) 143
blood tests 163
blood transfusion/exchange transfusion 113
BMPR2 gene 62, 63–4, 70, 163
BMPR2 mutation carriers, genetic testing for 64
bosentan 70, 215
  arrhythmias 208
  chronic thromboembolic pulmonary hypertension (CTEPH) 149
  drug interactions 219
  idiopathic pulmonary fibrosis 129
  portopulmonary hypertension (POPH) 96
  specific therapies 215, 218, 217–216
brain natriuretic peptide (BNP) 139, 163
bridging therapy 149

C

calcium channel blockers (CCBs) 200, 212–13, 218
  acute vasodilator testing 194
  combination therapy 220
  pregnancy and contraception 205
  systemic sclerosis/ scleroderma (SSc) 77
  in vasodilator positive patients 212
carbamazepine 219
cardiac catheterization 186
  complications of right heart catheterization (RHC) using balloon catheters 187
  conditions to exclude during right heart catheterization (RHC) 191
  constriction and restriction 191–2
  coronary angiography 186

data recorded at right heart catheterization (RHC) and technique 189, 190
Fick principle 189
lung disease 193
normal right heart catheterization (RHC) values 187
prognostic data from right heart catheterization (RHC) 191
right heart catheterization (RHC) 186
shunting 191
Swan-Ganz catheterization technique 187
cardiac index 51
cardiac magnetic resonance imaging (CMR) 171–2
cardiac shunts *see* congenital systemic-to-pulmonary cardiac shunts
cardiopulmonary exercise testing (CPET) 184
catheters/catheterization:
  Swan-Ganz 186–7
  ureteric 4
  see also cardiac catheterization; right heart catheterization
CD4+ cells 88
cellular factors in pulmonary artery remodelling 47
central nervous system disease 84
cercariae 106
chemotherapeutic agents 72
chest crisis, acute 113
chest X-ray 138, 161
chorionic villus sampling 64
chronic haemolytic anaemias 109–115
  acute chest crisis 113
  aplastic crisis 112
  diagnosis of sickle cell disease 110
  haemolytic crises 111
  hydroxyurea 114
  long-term management of sickle cell disease 114
  management of sickle cell crisis 112
  pathophysiology of sickle cell disease 110, 114
  prevalence of PH in sickle cell disease 114
  prevention of sickle cell disease 115
  proposed mechanisms in sickle cell disease 114

sickle cell disease 110
  sickling and nitric oxide (NO) resistance 113
  splenic sequestration crises 112
  thrombotic crises 111
  treatment of haemoglobino-pathies 115
  vaso-occlusive crises 111
chronic heart failure 67
chronic obstructive pulmonary disease (COPD) 14, 67, 211
chronic thromboembolic disease (CTED) 78, 148, 168
chronic thromboembolic pulmonary hypertension (CTEPH) 13, 43, 67, 134, 136, 147–151
  anticoagulation 148, 210
  diagnosis and investigations 158
  diagnostic algorithm 159–60
  epidemiology 66
  functional class after pulmonary endarterectomy (PEA) 150
  haemodynamic changes after pulmonary endarterectomy (PEA) 150
  indications for pulmonary endarterectomy (PEA) 150
  management 199, 202
  medical treatment for inoperable type 148
  pathology 36
  perioperative mortality 150
  pulmonary angiography and magnetic resonance imaging 167, 169–70
  pulmonary endarterectomy (PEA) 149
  specific therapies 214
  surgical technique 150
  survival rates 150
  symptoms 157
  and systemic lupus erythematosus (SLE) 85
  ventilation/perfusion (V/Q) lung scan 164
cigarette smoking 72
clexane 148
clinical monitoring 200–201

clinical psychologists 199
cocaine 72
combination therapy 149,
    212, 220, 223
complex cyanotic congenital
    heart disease with
    pulmonary blood
    flow 101
complications 201
compression stockings
    and post-thrombotic
    syndrome (PTS) 144
computed tomography
    (CT) 192
  high resolution
    (HRCT) 166
  of pulmonary arteries
    (CTPA) 140, 167, 168
concentric and eccentric
    non-laminar intimal
    fibrosis (onion bulb
    lesions) 26
congenital heart disease
    (CHD) 66–7, 100, 171
  advanced therapies 212
  anticoagulation 210
  complex 67, 103
  complex cyanotic, with
    pulmonary blood
    flow 101
  diagnosis and
    investigations 194
  oxygen therapy 211
  specific therapies 215
congenital systemic-to-
    pulmonary cardiac
    shunts 99–104
  anatomical-
    pathophysiological
    classification 102
  classification of congenital
    heart disease
    anomalies 101
  congenital heart
    disease 100
  histology 104
  medical treatment 104
connective tissue disease
    (CTD) 20, 26, 42,
    46, 76
  advanced therapies
    212, 216
  clinical features 76
  diagnosis and
    investigations 157,
    166, 184, 194
  and endothelin receptor
    antagonists 215
  epidemiology 66
  genetic screening 64
  identification of causes 78
  immunology and antibody
    profiles 77

management 201
mixed (MCTD) 76
pathology 76
pregnancy and
    contraception 205
prevalence 76
prognosis 77
screening 76
specific therapies 212
vasodilator testing 77
consultation 199
continuity of care 199
contraception issues 72,
    203–4, 219
contrast venography 136
conventional invasive
    pulmonary
    angiography 169
coronary angiography
    56, 186
coronary artery disease
    (CAD) 77
coronary syndromes,
    acute 141
cyclophosphamide 80,
    83–4, 129
cyclosporine 219
CYP2C9 inhibitors 219
CYP3A4 inhibitors 90, 219
cytokines 89

D

dabigatran etexilate
    143, 148
dalteparin 141
Dana Point (2008) clinical
    classification 16, 126
D-dimer testing 136
deep vein thrombosis
    (DVT) 43, 134, 143
  acute pulmonary
    embolism 138
  of the arm 144
  clinical features 135
  contrast venography 136
  duplex ultrasonography
    (DU) 136
  pathophysiology 135
  prevention 144
  and pulmonary embolism
    (PE) 141
  screening 144
  thrombolytic therapy 141
  treatment 141
definition of pulmonary
    hypertension/pulmonary
    arterial hypertension 8
dermatomyositis 76, 86
dexfenfluramine 5
diagnosis and
    investigations 66,
    155–194, 200

acute vasodilator testing
    (VT) 194
blood tests 163
cardiac magnetic
    resonance imaging
    (CMR) 171–2
cardiopulmonary exercise
    testing (CPET) 184
chest X-ray 161
conventional invasive
    pulmonary
    angiography 169
diagnostic algorithm 159
diagnostic tests 160
Doppler echocardio-
    graphy 173, 175
echocardiography 173
electrocardiogram
    (ECG) 161
exercise testing for
    ischaemic heart
    disease 185
genetic testing 163
high resolution computed
    tomography
    (HRCT) 166
lung function tests 162
magnetic resonance
    (MR) pulmonary
    angiography 170
non-invasive exercise
    testing 184
prognostic markers of
    right ventricular failure
    and death 156
pulmonary angiography
    and magnetic
    resonance
    scanning 167
  rationale 212
  screening 174
signs of associated
    disease 157–8
6MWD 184
6MWT 158
symptoms 156
ventilation/perfusion
    (V/Q) lung
    scan 164–5
World Health
    Organization
    (WHO) functional
    classification 157
  see also cardiac
    catheterization;
    echocardiographic
    assessment of right
    ventricle
diastolic function 180
digitalis 4
digoxin 149, 211
dihydropyridine 213
diltiazem 194, 205, 213

diuretics 149, 201, 205, 210
Doppler
    echocardiography 173,
    175, 192
dose-response
    characteristics of specific
    drugs 217
drug interactions with
    targeted therapies 219
drugs and toxins 72
    definite risk factors 72
    likely risk factors 72
    possible risk factors 72
    unlikely risk factors 72
drug trials, problems in
    conducting 222
duplex ultrasonography
    (DU) 136

E

eccentricity index 182
echocardiographic
    assessment of right
    ventricle (RV) 176
    diastolic function 180
    features of PH 181
    geometric measurement
    of right ventricular
    function 177
    left heart disease 182–3
    myocardial performance
    index (MPI; Tei
    index) 178
    normal RV
    measurements 181
    pericardial effusion 176
    stress
    echocardiography 183
    3D echocardiography 183
    tricuspid annular plane
    systolic excursion
    (TAPSE) 179
echocardiography 66, 173
    Doppler 173, 175, 192
    transthoracic and
    transoesophageal 139
    see also echocardiographic
    assessment
edoxaban 148
Eisenmenger's
    syndrome 67, 212,
    215, 225
elective surgery 207
electrocardiogram
    (ECG) 161
    acute pulmonary
    embolism (PE) 138
    in right heart disease 52
embolic obstruction 169
emphysema 34
end of life issues 199
endoglin (ENG) 62–3

endothelin 40, 42
endothelin pathway 212
endothelin receptor
    antagonists (ERAs) 40,
    201, 212, 215
    chronic thromboembolic
    pulmonary
    hypertension
    (CTEPH) 149
    combination therapy 220
    connective tissue
    disease 215
    human immunodeficiency
    virus (HIV) 90
    pregnancy and
    contraception 203–5
    specific therapies 214–15
    systemic sclerosis/
    scleroderma (SSc) 80
endothelin receptors 214
end systolic pressure
    volume relationships
    (ESPVR) assessments 54
enoxaparin 141
epidemiology 65–68
    congenital heart
    disease 67
    group 2: left heart
    disease 67
    group 3: lung diseases
    with or without
    hypoxaemia 67
    group 4: chronic
    thromboembolic PH
    (CTEPH) 67
    group 5: unclear and/
    or multifactorial
    mechanisms 67
    prevalence of PAH in
    subgroups 68
    pulmonary veno-occlusive
    disease (PVOD) and/
    or pulmonary capillary
    haemangiomatosis
    (PCH) 70
epidermal growth factor
    (EGF) 46
epidural anaesthesia 207
epoprostenol 194, 213,
    217–18
    drug trials 223
    portal hypertension 97
Epstein-Barr virus 47
erythromycin 219
Europe 210
exercise 202
    endpoints, interpretation
    of 222
    testing for ischaemic heart
    disease 185
    testing, non-invasive 184
    see also 6MWD
experimental drugs 223

F

factor VIII protein 43
factor Xa inhibitors 141,
    143, 148
familial PAH 20, 63, 66, 70
fenfluramine 5, 72
fibrotic and proliferative
    vascular lesions 26
Fick formula 189
Fick principle 189
fitness to fly testing 206
fluconazole 219
folic acid 112
fondaparinux 141–2
future study designs and
    endpoints 223–4

G

gadolinium
    enhancement 56
general anaesthesia 207
general health issues 201
genetic testing 63–4, 163
    during pregnancy for
    BMPR2 mutation
    carriers 64
    in heritable PAH 64
genomics 63
glib 219
goal directed therapy 221
grapefruit juice 219
growth factors 46, 89

H

haemodynamic
    classification 11
haemodynamic dangers of
    pregnancy 204
haemodynamics 192
haemoglobinopathies 115
haemolytic anaemias see
    chronic haemolytic
    anaemias
haemolytic crises 111
haemorrhagic telangiectasia,
    hereditary (HHT) 62–3
haemosiderin deposits 27
Hampton's hump 161
heart failure:
    chronic 67
    see also right heart
    failure
heat and right ventricle
    preload 202
heparin 141
    -induced thrombo-
    cytopaenia 143
    unfractionated
    (UFH) 141–2
hepatitis C 47

hereditary haemorrhagic telangiectasia (HHT) 62–3
hereditary pulmonary arterial hypertension (HPAH) 62, 63, 64
hereditary thrombophilia 43
high resolution computed tomography (HRCT) 166
history of pulmonary hypertension and circulation 4
holistic management and support 198
Hughes syndrome 83
human immunodeficiency virus (HIV) 46–7, 87–91
  advanced therapies 212
  anticoagulation 210
  arrhythmias 208
  diagnosis and investigations 90, 158, 194
  endothelin receptor antagonists (ERAs) 90
  epidemiology and management 66, 70, 88–9
  prognosis 90
  prostanoids 91
  and pulmonary hypertension 89
  sildenafil 90
  stages of infection 88
  virology and immunology 88
  warfarin 91
hydroxychloroquine 83–4
hydroxyurea 114
hypertrophy 26
  medial 26
hypoxaemia 34
hypoxia 66

I

idiopathic PAH 62, 63
  advanced therapies 213–14, 215
  anticoagulation 210
  diagnosis and investgations 161, 166–7, 184, 194
  drugs and toxins 72
  epidemiology 66, 70
  inflammation 198
  multidisciplinary approach 198
  pathology 26

pregnancy and contraception 205
prognosis 20
  surgical interventions 225
idiopathic pulmonary fibrosis (IPF) 127–8
  usual interstitial pneumonia (UIP) 126–8
idrabiotaparinux 148
iloprost 194, 214, 218
immunoglobulin G (IgG) 76
immunosuppression 80, 85, 129, 227
incentive spirometry 113
infection risk and vaccination 206
inflammation 46, 89
inlet portion 50
interferon gamma–1b 129
interferon, topical 86
interstitial lung disease (ILD) 126, 127, 129
  epidemiology 67
  high resolution computed tomography (HRCT) 166
  management 200
interstitial pulmonary fibrosis (IPF)
  treatment 129
intravascular thrombosis 26
invasive pulmonary angiography, conventional 169
investigations see diagnosis and investigations
ischaemic heart disease 185

J

joint clinics 198

K

ketoconazole 219

L

left heart disease 42, 56, 67
  diagnosis and investigations 159, 182–3
  epidemiology 66
  haemodynamics and treatment approaches 119–121
  haemodynamics and treatment approaches:
    diagnosis of post-capillary pulmonary hypertension 121

disproportionate post-capillary pulmonary hypertension 120
    presentation of post-capillary PH 120
    treatment of post-capillary PH 121
  pathology 32
  and post-capillary PH 13, 14
left-sided inflow obstruction 101
left-to-right shunts due to volume and pressure loading of pulmonary vasculature 101
left ventricle 50, 53–4
left ventricular hypertrophy 161
lepirudin (Refludan®) 143
lesions:
  arterial 26
  concentric and eccentric non-laminar intimal fibrosis (onion bulb) 26
  fibrotic and proliferative vascular 26
  plexiform 26, 27, 46
  producing left-to-right shunts due to volume and pressure loading of pulmonary vasculature 101
  vasculitic 27
  venous 27
lifestyle factors 206, 208
liver disease, chronic 158
liver transplantation 96
local anaesthesia 207
low-molecular-weight heparin (LMWH) 205, 210
  acute pulmonary embolism 141–2
  chronic thromboembolic pulmonary hypertension (CTEPH) 148
L-tryptophan 72
lung disease 13, 66, 125–130, 193
  and/or hypoxaemia 67
  and/or hypoxia 34, 42
  classification of interstitial lung disease (ILD) 129
  clinical features suggestive of interstitial lung disease (ILD) 127
  diagnosis of PH in idiopathic pulmonary fibrosis (IPF) 128

lung disease (cont.)
diagnostic criteria for idiopathic pulmonary fibrosis (IPF) (usual interstitial pneumonia (UIP)) 126–8
histology of idiopathic pulmonary fibrosis (IPF) 127
interstitial lung disease (ILD) and systemic sclerosis or scleroderma (SSc) 129
interstitial pulmonary fibrosis (IPF) treatment 129
non-specific interstitial pneumonia (NSIP) 130
treatment of interstitial lung disease (ILD) 129
lung fibrosis 34, 78–77
lung function testing 42, 66, 162
lung samples 26
lung windows 167–8
lupus anticoagulant 43
lupus nephritis 84

M

magnetic resonance imaging (MRI) 192
cardiac (CMR) 171–2
pulmonary angiography 170
scanning 167
management 197–208
aims of treatment 198
arrhythmias, atrial 208
arrhythmias, ventricular 208
consultation 199
continuity of care 199
contraception 203–4
elective surgery 207
end of life issues 199
fitness to fly testing 206
heat and right ventricle preload 202
holistic management and support 198
infection risk and vaccination 206
issues to be addressed in clinic 200
lifestyle issues 206
multidisciplinary multispecialty clinics 198
patient expectations, hopes and fears 198
pregnancy 204

rehabilitation and exercise 202
supportive measures 202
travel 206
manometers 4
matrix metalloproteases 40
mean pulmonary artery pressure (mPAP):
during exercise 9
normal value 9
significance of 21–24mmHg 9
medial hypertrophy 26
mepacrine 84
methamphetamines 72
methotrexate 83
miricidia 106
mitral valve disease 67
mortality rates 20, 204–5, 207
multidisciplinary multispecialty approach/ clinics 198, 207
mycophenolate 83, 129
mycophenolate mofetil 84
myocardial fibrosis 77–78
myocardial ischaemia 77
myocardial performance index (MPI; Tei index) 54, 178

N

N-acetylcysteine 129
natural history 20
nicorandil 216–17, 219
nifedipine 194, 205, 213
nitrates 216–17, 219
nitric oxide (NO) 40, 194
pathway 212
resistance and sickling 113
non-laminar intimal fibrosis, concentric and eccentric (onion bulb lesions) 26
non-specific interstitial pneumonia (NSIP) 127, 130
non-steroidal anti-inflammatory drugs (NSAIDs) 83
non-targeted therapy 149
N-terminal fragment of pro-brain natriuretic peptide (NT-proBNP) 163
nurse specialists 199

O

oedema:
peripheral 200
pulmonary 70, 161
oestrogen 72

oral contraceptives 72, 219
outflow or infundibular portion 50
'out of proportion' PH 14, 42, 193
outreach clinics 200
over-the-counter drugs 208
oxygen therapy 34, 112–13, 211
pregnancy and contraception 205
and travelling 206

P

palliative care 201
patent ductus arteriosus (PDA) 67, 100
pathobiology 40
pathogenetic pathways 212
pathology 25–28
arterial lesions 26
chronic thromboembolic pulmonary hypertension (CTEPH) 36
left heart disease 32
lung diseases and/or hypoxia 34
lung samples 26
plexiform lesions 26–7
pulmonary capillary haemangiomatosis (PCH) 30
pulmonary veno-occlusive disease (PVOD) 30
unclear and/or multifactorial mechanisms 38
vasculitic lesions 27
venous lesions 27
pathophysiology 41–43
group 2: left heart disease 42
group 3: lung diseases and/or hypoxia 42
group 4: chronic thromboembolic pulmonary hypertension (CTEPH) 43
patient expectations, hopes and fears, management of 198
penicillin 112
pericardial effusion 176, 177
peripheral oedema 200
pharmacists 199
phenobarbital 219
phentermine/fenfluramine 5
phenylpropanolamine 72
phenytoin 219

phlegmasia cerulea dolens 145
phosphodiesterase-5 inhibitors 32, 40, 216–17
   combination therapy 220
   dose-response characteristics 217
   drug interactions 219
   pathogenetic pathways 212
   portopulmonary hypertension (POPH) 96
   pregnancy and contraception 204–5
   sildenafil 216
   systemic sclerosis/ scleroderma (SSc) 80
   tadalafil 217
physicians with specialist knowledge of PH 198
physiological changes associated with pregnancy, labour and delivery 204
pimecrolimus 83
platelet-derived growth factor (PDGF) 46, 89
plexiform lesions 26, 27, 46
polymyositis 76, 86
portal/portopulmonary hypertension (POPH) 20, 26, 93–97
   anticoagulation 210
   arrhythmias 208
   classification 94
   clinical presentation 95
   diagnosis and investigations 95, 194
   haemodynamics 95
   medical treatment 96
   pathophysiology 94
   prognosis 97
   screening 95
post-capillary PH 78
   'out of proportion' 14, 42
   see also left heart disease
post-thrombotic syndrome (PTS) 134, 136, 144
post-transplant immunosuppressive treatment 227
post-tricuspid shunts, simple 103
praziquantel 107
prednisolone 83, 129
pregnancy 204
   termination 204

and venous thromboembolism (VTE) 141, 145
pre-implantation genetic diagnosis 64
pressure loaded right ventricle 49–58
   anatomy 50
   chest X-ray imaging 53
   echocardiography 54, 55
   electrocardiogram (ECG) in right heart disease 52
   invasive assessment 58
   left heart disease and PH 56
   magnetic resonance imaging (MRI) 56–7
   pathophysiology 50
pre-tricuspid shunts, simple 102
procedures and treatments, classes of recommendations for 218
prognosis 20
proliferative pulmonary vasculopathy 78
prostacyclin pathway 212
prostacyclins 40, 149, 217
prostaglandins 210
prostanoids 201, 210, 217
   combination therapy 220
   human immunodeficiency virus (HIV) 91
   pathogenetic pathways 212
   portopulmonary hypertension (POPH) 96–7
   pregnancy and contraception 204–5
   pulmonary veno-occlusive disease and/or pulmonary capillary haemangiomatosis 70
   systemic sclerosis/ scleroderma (SSc) 80
protease inhibitors 216, 219
psychological problems 201
pulmonary angiography 167
   conventional invasive 169
   magnetic resonance 170
pulmonary arterial pressure tracing 8
pulmonary arteries of veins, anomalies of 101
pulmonary arteriolar vasoconstriction/ remodelling 14
pulmonary arteriovenous malformations 169

pulmonary artery occlusion pressure (PAOP) tracing 11–13
pulmonary artery vascular remodelling 47
pulmonary capillary haemangiomatosis (PCH) pathology 30
pulmonary capillary wedge pressure 14
pulmonary embolectomy 142
pulmonary embolism (PE) 135–6, 141
   and chronic thromboembolic pulmonary hypertension (CTEPH) 148
   diagnosis and investigations 157, 170
   see also acute pulmonary embolism
pulmonary endarterectomy (PEA) 149
   functional class 150
   haemodynamic changes 150
   indications for 150
pulmonary fibrosis 76, 78–9
   interstitial (IPF) 129
   see also idiopathic pulmonary fibrosis
pulmonary function testing 42, 66, 162
pulmonary oedema 70, 161
pulmonary vascular resistance (PVR) 10
pulmonary vasculopathy 14, 66
pulmonary vasodilators 77, 148, 207
pulmonary veno-occlusive disease (PVOD) 27, 30, 78, 80
   and/or pulmonary capillary haemangiomatosis (PCH) 70
   diagnosis and investigations 157, 166
   management 199
   pathology 30
   specific therapies 212

R

radiofrequency ablation 208
radiologists 199
rapeseed oil 72
rehabilitation 202
renal transplantation 83
respiratory failure 67
rheumatoid arthritis 76

rheumatoid factor
(RhF) 76–7
rifampicin 219
right atrial pressure 51
right heart catheterization
(RHC):
and systemic sclerosis or
scleroderma (SSc) 77
see also cardiac
catheterization
right heart disease and
electrocardiogram
(ECG) 52
right heart failure 70,
202, 210
right ventricle/ventricular:
death and prognostic
markers 156
failure 77, 156
function 78
hypertrophy 161
outflow tract
(RVOT) 177
preload and heat 202
systolic pressure
(TRV) 173
see also echocardiographic
assessment of right
ventricle; pressure
loaded right ventricle
ritonavir 90, 219
rivaroxaban 143, 148

S

St John's wort 72, 219
Schirmer's test 86
schistosomiasis 105–107
chronic 106–7
clinical features 107
diagnosis 106
parasite life cycle 106
pathophysiology 107
treatment 107
schistosomula 106
screening 20
sedatives 207
selective serotonin
reuptake inhibitors
(SSRIs) 72, 211
serotonin (5-HT) and
serotonin transporter
(5-HTT) 47–46
severe PAH 202
shared care 200
shunting 191
sickle cell disease see
chronic haemolytic
anaemias
sildenafil 214, 216–18
chronic thromboembolic
pulmonary hypertension
(CTEPH) 149

drug interactions 219
drug trials 223
human immunodeficiency
virus (HIV) 90
interstitial lung disease
(ILD) 129
pulmonary veno-occlusive
disease (PVOD) and/
or pulmonary capillary
haemangiomatosis
(PCH) 70
sitaxsentan 215–16
6MWD (6 minute walk
distance) 184, 220, 222,
223–4
6MWT (6 minute walk
test) 158
Sjögren's syndrome 76, 86
skin rashes 83
social problems 201
social workers 199
specific therapies 209–228
anticoagulation 212
antidepressants 211
classes of
recommendations
for procedures and
treatments 218
combination therapy 220
digoxin 211
diuretics 210
drug interactions with
PAH-targeted
therapies 219
drug trials, problems in
conducting 222
oxygen 211
supportive medical
therapies 210
see also advanced
therapies; surgical
interventions
spironolactone 211
splenic sequestration
crises 112
statins 219
steroids 80
low-dose 83
oral 129
topical 83
strain and strain-rate
assessments 54
subgroups, prevalence
of pulmonary arterial
hypertension in 68
sun-blockers 83
supportive medical
therapies 202, 210
surgical interventions 225
atrial septostomy 225
transplantation 226
survival data 20, 223, 228
survivin 47

Swan-Ganz catheterization
technique 186–7
S-wave velocity 180
systemic lupus
erythematosus (SLE) 76,
81, 205
activity monitoring 82
antiphospholipid
syndrome (APS) 82
arthralgia and skin
rashes 83
central nervous system
disease 84
and chronic
thromboembolic
pulmonary
hypertension
(CTEPH) 85
diagnosis 81
lupus nephritis 84
management 85
organ complications 82
pathobiology 81
physical signs 82
prevalence and
epidemiology 81
prognosis 84
and pulmonary
hypertension 84
treatment 83
systemic sclerosis or
scleroderma (SSc) 20,
76, 79, 129
advanced therapies 213,
215, 217
anticoagulation 210
causes 78
clinical features 76
diagnosis and
investigations 77, 158
diffuse 79–80
epidemiology and
management 66,
70, 80
immunological testing 80
limited 79
mechanisms of PH 78
and non-specific interstitial
pneumonia 130
prognosis 77–78
pulmonary function tests
(PFTs) 80
vasodilator testing 77
systemic-to-pulmonary
cardiac shunts
see congenital
systemic-to-pulmonary
cardiac shunts

T

tacrolimus 83
tadalafil 217–18

targeted therapies 97, 200, 206, 218
tecarfarin 148
tenascin 40
therapeutic advances in treatment 212
thoracic outlet syndrome 144
three-dimensional echo 54
thrombin inhibitors, direct 143, 148
thrombocytopaenia, heparin-induced 143
thromboembolic pulmonary hypertension see chronic thromboembolic pulmonary hypertension
thromboendarterectomy 85
thrombolysis 142, 144
thrombolytic therapy for deep vein thrombosis (DVT) 141
thrombophilia, hereditary 43
thrombosis 47
  in situ 43
  intravascular 26
thrombotic crises 111
thromboxane A2 40
tinzaparin 141
tissue plasminogen activator (rtPA) 142
toxins see drugs and toxins
trabecular portion 50
transplantation 83, 96, 226
transpulmonary pressure gradient (TPG) 14
travel 206
treatment rationale 212
trematode worms 106
treprostinil 214, 217–18
tricuspid annular plane systolic excursion (TAPSE) 54, 179
tricuspid annulus velocity 54, 180
troponins 139, 163
two-dimensional echo 192

U

unclear and/or multifactorial mechanisms 13, 38, 67
  see also idiopathic

unfractionated heparin (UFH) 141–2
United States 210
  Genetics Information Nondiscrimination Act (2008) 63
ureteric catheters 4
usual interstitial pneumonia (UIP) 126–8

V

vascular endothelial growth factor (VEGF) 46, 89
vasculitic lesions 27
vasculitis 169
vasoactive intestinal polypeptide (VIP) 40
vasoconstrictors 206
vasodilators:
  drug trials 223
  pulmonary 77, 148, 207
  vasodilator testing (VT) 70, 77, 194
vaso-occlusive crises 111
vector velocity imaging 54
vena caval interruption 142
venous lesions 27
venous thromboembolism (VTE) 43, 133–136, 141, 143
  acute 67
  and chronic thromboembolic pulmonary hypertension (CTEPH) 148
  clinical features of deep vein thrombosis (DVT) 135
  contrast venography 136
  D-dimer testing 136
  deep vein thrombosis (DVT) 135
  duplex ultrasonography (DU) 136
  during pregnancy 141
  investigations 136
  and long-term anticoagulation 144

pathophysiology and natural history 135
and pregnancy 145
prevalence 134
prevention 144
pulmonary embolism (PE) 135, 136
risk factors 134
screening 144
ventilation/perfusion scanning 140, 164–5
ventricular septal defects (VSDs) 67, 100
verapamil 213
viral and other infectious factors 47
volume and pressure loading of pulmonary vasculature 101

W

warfarin 210, 212
  acute pulmonary embolism 143
  deep vein thrombosis (DVT) 141
  drug interactions 219
  human immunodeficiency virus (HIV) 91
  infection risk and vaccination 206
  systemic lupus erythematosus 83, 85
Westermark's sign of transradiancy 161
World Health Organization functional classes I – IV 20, 198, 215, 218
  chronic thromboembolic PH 149
  diagnosis and investigations 156, 194
  human immunodeficiency virus (HIV) 90
  travel 206

X

X-ray, chest 138, 161